AVASTIN

The Miracle Drug Redefining Hope for Cancer Patients

By

ROBERT D. SHARP

Table of Contents

Abstract

Avastin: The Miracle Drug Redefining Hope for Cancer Patients" is an exploration of the groundbreaking impact of Avastin (bevacizumab) in the realm of cancer treatment. This abstract delves into the drug's innovative mechanism of action, its notable successes, and the newfound hope it offers to cancer patients, revolutionizing the landscape of oncology care.

CHAPTER 1

**The Quest for a Cancer Miracle
Introduction to the challenges of cancer
treatment and the search for innovative
solutions.**

The Mysteries of Cancer

Cancer is more than just a sickness; it's a dynamic, multifaceted enemy. It takes on multiple shapes and is not restricted by a single set of laws. Every kind of cancer, including pancreatic and breast cancer, has different traits and requires a customized strategy. The fact that this disease can affect any area of the body adds to its complexity and is a significant challenge for medical practitioners.

Present-Day Treatment Approaches

Several important therapy techniques have been created by the medical profession in the continuous fight against cancer. When feasible, surgery has proven beneficial in the removal of localized tumors. High-energy radiation is used in radiation treatment to kill cancer cells. Numerous lives have been saved by chemotherapy, which uses medications to target and kill cancer cells that divide quickly. Using the body's immune system to combat cancer, immunotherapy has become a more viable strategy in recent times.

Although many patients' lives have been prolonged and enhanced by these treatments, they are not without drawbacks. Surgery can have both physical and psychological side effects, and it may not always be possible. Chemotherapy and radiation, although very beneficial, can have severe side effects. To reduce these side effects, increase treatment precision, and eventually improve patient outcomes, creative solutions are sought after.

The Human Price

The effects of cancer are felt well outside of hospital rooms and research facilities. It is incredibly intimate and fundamentally human. It causes misery and suffering, upends lives, and can have the most tragic results. A cancer diagnosis has a cascading effect on communities, families, and friends. The toll that it takes on patients and their loved ones, both physically and emotionally, highlights how urgently better therapies are needed.

Creativity and Hope

An unwavering feeling of hope fuels the "quest for a cancer miracle". It is the conviction that, in spite of the enormous obstacles, we can discover fresh approaches to treating this illness. Globally, scientists, doctors, and patients are united in the belief that science, ingenuity, and human spirit can transcend the seemingly insurmountable challenges presented by cancer.

We shall read about the lives of those who have devoted themselves to this goal as we travel through the pages of this book. We will learn about the scientific discoveries, unwavering tenacity, and teamwork that have brought us this close to achieving a cancer miracle. The road ahead is paved with obstacles and victories, failures and discoveries, but most of all, it is lit by the unflinching conviction that a better future is not just feasible, but getting closer for cancer patients.

Of course, let's go into more detail in Chapter 1: The Search for a Cancer Miracle, which provides an overview of the difficulties associated with treating cancer and suggests some creative solutions.

The Mysteries of Cancer

Cancer is a puzzle with many complex answers. It does not confine itself to a single entity, but rather manifests itself in a variety of ways, each with distinct traits, behaviors, and reactions to various treatments. For example, breast cancer is a broad category that includes multiple subtypes, such as hormone receptor-positive and triple-negative breast cancer, each of which needs a distinct approach. Likewise, leukemia and lymphoma are blood cell-derived diseases that require different treatment strategies due to their unique characteristics.

Cancer's complexity stems from both its wide range of expressions and its ability to change and adapt. In order to resist the body's defenses and conventional therapies, cancer cells frequently undergo mutations and develop evasion mechanisms. Because of its versatility, it is a very difficult opponent that requires a constantly changing strategy.

Present-Day Treatment Approaches

The medical community has created a toolbox of cancer treatment choices throughout the years, each having a specific role to play in the fight against this powerful foe.

Surgery: The treatment of cancer has greatly benefited from surgery. The goal is to eradicate localized tumors as much as possible. Nevertheless, not all malignancies can be treated surgically, and when it can, the procedure might have serious negative psychological and physical effects.

High-energy radiation beams are used in radiation treatment to target and kill cancer cells. It's especially helpful when the cancer is confined and incurable. Although it has been an important component of cancer treatment, it frequently causes side effects and must be administered precisely.

Chemotherapy: Using strong medications to target and destroy cancer cells that divide quickly is known as chemotherapy. It has saved countless lives as a staple of cancer treatment for many years. However, side effects from chemotherapy are well-known and can include everything from nausea and hair loss to compromised immune system function.

Immunotherapy: A relatively new treatment option for cancer is immunotherapy. It makes use of the immune system of the body to locate and eliminate cancer cells. Although this method isn't always successful, it has demonstrated amazing potential in some cancer cases.

These treatments are not without their drawbacks, despite the fact that they have significantly improved the prognosis for cancer patients. Genetic variations, cancer kind, and stage are some of the reasons that may restrict its effectiveness. Furthermore, these therapies frequently come with a unique set of difficulties and adverse effects. Therefore, the drive to find novel solutions stems from a desire to maximize the positive effects of these treatments on patients' quality of life while simultaneously improving their accuracy and efficacy.

The Human Price

There is the very human aspect of suffering in addition to the scientific difficulties of cancer treatment. Cancer upends lives, causes mental and physical suffering, and, in the worst situations, results in the death of loved ones. Feelings of anxiety, uneasiness, and discomfort are frequently experienced following a cancer diagnosis. It may have an adverse effect on the sufferer as well as their friends, family, and community.

The human cost of cancer serves as a potent catalyst for reform. It highlights how urgent it is to develop better therapies that can lessen the misery brought on by this illness. This mission is evidence of the human race's collective compassion and the unwavering search for ways to reduce the toll that cancer takes on its victims.

Creativity and Hope

An unshakable feeling of hope drives the "quest for a cancer miracle". It is the conviction that we can come up with creative solutions to fight this illness, even in the face of enormous obstacles. Scientists, doctors, and patients everywhere believe that human spirit, ingenuity, and science can get over the seemingly insurmountable challenges that cancer presents.

We're going to take a journey through the lives of those who have devoted themselves to this pursuit in the pages that follow. We will explore the scientific discoveries, unwavering tenacity, and teamwork that have brought us this close to achieving a cancer miracle. The road ahead is paved with obstacles and victories, failures and discoveries, but most of all, it is lit by the unflinching conviction that a better future is not just feasible, but getting closer for cancer patients. The future chapters will shed light on how Avastin redefined that hope and changed the face of cancer treatment.

CHAPTER 2

**Avastin's Journey from Lab to Clinic
The development and approval process
of Avastin as a cancer treatment.
The process of developing and
approving Avastin as a treatment for
cancer.**

The Origin of a Lucrative Concept

Avastin's journey from the lab to the clinic is a tale of scientific inventiveness, perseverance, and resourcefulness. It all started with a very intriguing hypothesis: would it be possible to stop the growth and spread of cancer by blocking the process of angiogenesis, which is the formation of new blood vessels?

This theory gained popularity in the late 20th century when scientists like Dr. Judah Folkman started investigating the possibility that cancer tumors required blood flow in order to develop and thrive. The notion was groundbreaking; it proposed that one might effectively starve the tumor by stopping its angiogenesis.

Early Findings in the Lab

Early on in Avastin's research, significant discoveries in the lab were made. Vascular endothelial growth factor (VEGF) is a protein that has been identified by researchers as being essential to angiogenesis. It was discovered that VEGF, when overexpressed in tumors, played a major factor in the development of blood vessels feeding the tumor.

An important person on this path, Dr. Napoleone Ferrara, was essential in identifying and defining VEGF. His research served as a basis for the creation of Avastin. Finding the importance of VEGF and how it promotes cancer angiogenesis was a lightbulb moment in the search for innovative cancer therapies.

The Development and Clinical Trials of Avastin

The development of Avastin transitioned from laboratory experiments to clinical trials upon the identification of VEGF. The biotechnology business Genentech, which played a key role in the development of Avastin, started an exacting procedure of preclinical research and early-stage clinical trials. The purpose of these trials was to evaluate the safety, dosage, and possible efficacy of Avastin in patients with different kinds of cancer.

Avastin demonstrated encouraging outcomes as it advanced through clinical trials. Specifically, the medication showed promise in the treatment of colorectal cancer. The drug's development underwent a major sea change at this point since it was among the first anti-angiogenic drugs to demonstrate clinical effectiveness in cancer patients.

Regulatory Acceptance and Growth

Regulatory approval was the final step in the trip from lab to clinic. 2004 saw the U.S. Avastin is approved by the Food and Drug Administration

(FDA) to treat metastatic colorectal cancer. This was a turning point in the history of cancer therapy. From a brilliant concept in a lab, Avastin has become a medication with clinical validation.

The list of cancers for which Avastin is approved has grown over time to include glioblastoma multiforme, renal cell carcinoma, and non-small cell lung cancer. This increase in indications was a reflection of our increasing knowledge of the drug's potential benefits for individuals with a variety of cancer types.

Avastin's Persistent Effect

Avastin's path from laboratory to clinic serves as a testament to the efficacy of translational research, which converts discoveries made in the lab into real-world clinical uses. In addition to prolonging the lives of many cancer patients, Avastin has completely changed the way that cancer is treated. It is a prime example of how scientific advancement may upend long-standing beliefs and provide fresh hope in the fight against cancer.

The details of Avastin's action, its involvement in different types of cancer, and the true tales of people whose lives have been impacted by this ground-breaking treatment will all be covered in the upcoming chapters. The story of Avastin's path is motivational and shows what can happen when science, creativity, and willpower come together to significantly impact the field of oncology.

Of course, let's take a closer look at Avastin's Journey from Lab to Clinic, which details the medication's development and approval process for the treatment of cancer.

The Origin of a Lucrative Concept

The idea that it might be possible to successfully stop the growth and spread of cancer by preventing the production of new blood vessels, a process known as angiogenesis, was the foundation of the Avastin adventure. A trailblazer in the profession, Dr. Judah Folkman was instrumental in presenting this revolutionary concept. Folkman's theory refuted accepted knowledge and sparked an idea that eventually resulted in the development of Avastin.

The knowledge that cancer tumors needed a network of blood arteries to supply them with nutrition and oxygen in order to grow and thrive was at the core of this theory. It may have been possible to "starve" the tumor by blocking this angiogenesis process, halting its spread and metastasis. This concept had far-reaching consequences and opened up a new avenue for the treatment of cancer.

Early Findings in the Lab

New findings in the lab throughout the early stages of Avastin's research contributed to our understanding of angiogenesis and its involvement in cancer. Inspired by Dr. Folkman's vision, scientists from all around the world investigated the complex mechanisms of angiogenesis.

The identification of vascular endothelial growth factor (VEGF) as a critical component in facilitating the development of new blood vessels was one important finding. It was discovered that VEGF, which is overexpressed in tumors, is a key factor in the development of blood vessels that supply the tumor. This discovery marked a sea change since it identified a precise area that needed to be addressed.

An important character in this story, Dr. Napoleone Ferrara, contributed a lot to the description of VEGF. His research was crucial in setting the stage for the creation of Avastin, a drug that binds to VEGF to block its function. This information marked a major advancement in the search for potent anti-angiogenic treatments.

The Development and Clinical Trials of Avastin

While translating lab findings into clinical practice is a difficult task, Genentech, the biotechnology company leading the way in Avastin's research, was committed to overcoming this obstacle. Preclinical testing and early-phase clinical trials were two of the rigorous processes involved in moving a treatment from the lab to the clinic.

The purpose of these trials was to evaluate Avastin's safety, ideal dosage, and possible efficacy in patients with different kinds of cancer. The outcomes were encouraging, especially in light of colorectal cancer. Avastin gave many patients new hope and a longer life expectancy. Being among the first anti-angiogenic drugs to show actual therapeutic benefit in cancer patients, this was a major turning point in the development of Avastin.

Regulatory Acceptance and Growth

Regulatory approval marked the happy culmination of the journey from lab to clinic. 2004 saw the U.S. Avastin has been approved by the Food and Drug Administration (FDA) to treat metastatic colorectal cancer. With this choice, Avastin became a scientifically validated medicine, a significant milestone in the history of cancer treatment.

Avastin's approval for different cancer types grew over time, indicating its adaptability and potential to help patients. The medicine was approved for the treatment of non-small cell lung cancer, glioblastoma multiforme, and renal cell carcinoma. This indicates that knowledge about the drug's effectiveness and effects on many cancer types is expanding.

Avastin's Persistent Effect

The path taken by Avastin from the lab to the clinic serves as an example of the effectiveness of translational research, which converts novel findings from the laboratory into useful therapeutic uses. In addition to saving the lives of many cancer patients, avastin has completely changed the way that cancer is treated. Its accomplishments demonstrate how scientific innovation has the power to upend long-held beliefs and provide fresh hope in the fight against cancer.

The details of Avastin's mode of action, its function in different forms of cancer, and the inspiring true experiences of patients whose lives have been significantly impacted by this ground-breaking treatment will all be covered in greater detail in the upcoming chapters. Avastin's story serves as an uplifting example of what happens when ingenuity, research, and steadfast resolve come together to significantly impact the field of oncology.

CHAPTER 3

Understanding Cancer: The Enemy Within Exploring the basics of cancer biology and the need for targeted therapies.

Cancer's Causes

Understanding the biology of cancer is a prerequisite to appreciating the significance of targeted medicines such as Avastin. Cancer is a phrase used to describe a group of diseases in which abnormal cells develop and spread uncontrollably. It does not refer to a specific disease. These cells start to evade the body's normal regulatory processes due to genetic abnormalities or environmental influences. As a result, cancerous tumors develop, which have the potential to invade surrounding tissues and, in more advanced stages, migrate to other parts of the body.

Understanding cancer starts at the cellular level. Trillions of cells make up our bodies, and each one has a distinct purpose and function. A fine balance between division, expansion, and programmed cell death controls these cells. Normal cells can become cancerous when this equilibrium is upset and genetic alterations mount up. These cells can proliferate quickly and uncontrollably, which can result in the development of a tumor.

The Intricacy of Cancer

The wide variety of cancer kinds, each with distinct features, highlights the complexity of cancer. Leukemia is not the same as colon cancer, nor is breast cancer the same as lung cancer. Furthermore, there may be several subtypes of a single type of cancer, each requiring a unique treatment strategy. A one-size-fits-all strategy is frequently insufficient, which emphasizes the need for medicines that can address the unique characteristics of each kind of cancer.

Genetic Mutations' Function

Genetic alterations are closely related to the development of cancer. Numerous things, like as exposure to carcinogens, mistakes in DNA replication, and inherited genetic predispositions, can result in these mutations.

Certain genetic mutations can start the chain of events that turns healthy cells into cancerous ones, even though not all genetic mutations cause cancer.

Developing successful treatments for cancer requires an understanding of its genetic foundations. Avastin is one example of a targeted therapy that is intended to disrupt particular biochemical pathways that are essential to the survival and proliferation of cancer cells. Targeted medicines seek to stop the disease's progression while protecting healthy cells by obstructing these pathways.

The Role of Targeted Treatments

Both malignant and healthy cells are frequently impacted by the traditional cancer treatment regimen, which consists of surgery, radiation therapy, and chemotherapy. Patients may experience severe side effects and a reduction in their quality of life as a result. The goal of increasing therapeutic precision gives rise to the necessity for tailored therapy.

The goal of targeted therapy is to specifically target the distinct molecular characteristics of cancer cells. They can mostly spare healthy cells from damage while blocking particular proteins or pathways that are necessary for the cancer to spread. This focused strategy may increase therapy efficacy while reducing adverse effects.

We will examine how Avastin, as a targeted therapy, uses our knowledge of cancer biology to cut off a tumor's blood supply in the upcoming chapters. It demonstrates the revolutionary potential of tailored medicines in the fight against cancer by doing this. The success of Avastin is not only a tribute to technological advancement but also to our growing comprehension of cancer as the enemy within and the necessity of specialized, accurate, and potent therapies to defeat it.

CHAPTER 4

Hope on the Horizon The initial excitement and promise of Avastin in the medical community.

the medical community's initial enthusiasm and optimism for Avastin.

A Glimmer of Hope

Few things in the medical field are as much anticipated as the introduction of a novel treatment. When Avastin was first introduced, it was just that—a ray of hope, showing the way toward a time when cancer could be treated with never-before-seen accuracy and potency.

Avastin's launch signaled a significant shift in the direction of cancer treatment, more so than the release of a new medication. When it finally arrived, it was like seeing a lighthouse in the distance—a symbol that a new, innovative, and hopeful era in medicine was approaching.

The Anti-Angiogenesis's Novelty

Avastin's unique anti-angiogenesis cancer treatment strategy was a major factor in the drug's initial buzz. This innovative approach differed from conventional techniques of directly targeting cancer cells. Rather, Avastin inhibited the growth of new blood vessels, which severed the tumor's essential blood supply.

Anti-angiogenesis posed a novel challenge because it may stop tumor growth while simultaneously preventing the development of new metastases. Basically, it presented a two-pronged approach to combating cancer, with potentially revolutionary results.

Initial Success Stories

Early success stories with Avastin emerged during clinical trials, especially in patients with metastatic colorectal cancer. These accounts provided concrete evidence that Avastin may live up to its promise, going beyond mere anecdotal evidence.

Avastin's effectiveness was demonstrated by patients who had better quality of life and longer survival times while on the medication. They themselves were hope-filled beacons, lighting the way for others who had fought the same illness and yearned for a successful cure.

Innovative Research and Experiments

There was more to the Avastin craze than just a few isolated success tales. The results of thorough clinical trials and studies supported it. Tests showing Avastin's adaptability and promise were conducted in a variety of cancer types, such as glioblastoma multiforme, breast cancer, and non-small cell lung cancer.

Every new investigation and clinical trial contributed to our growing knowledge of Avastin's potential and provided additional evidence of its efficacy. The outcomes kept the medical community excited and provided a glimpse of a future in which tailored treatments like Avastin will be essential in the battle against cancer.

Reorienting Viewpoints

The introduction of avastin changed the perception of cancer treatment. It brought about a paradigm change from focusing only on cancer cells to tackling the supporting cast, or the blood arteries that allowed tumors to grow. This shift in viewpoint highlighted the significance of individualized treatments based on the particulars of each patient's illness and opened up new avenues for cancer therapy.

Avastin was more than just a medication; it was a representation of optimism and proof of the medical community's unwavering search for novel treatments. It was the beginning of a new era in which cancer was no longer only an enemy but rather a task that could be accomplished with cunning, accuracy, and ultimately success.

We will delve more into Avastin's mechanisms of action, clinical uses, and the compelling patient stories that support its initial promise in the upcoming chapters as we continue to explore this journey. When Avastin first became known as a ray of hope, it was just the beginning of a journey that would change the face of cancer therapy and show patients how to live better lives.

CHAPTER 5

Unveiling the Mechanism: How Avastin Works Explaining the science behind Avastin's action against cancer.

describing the mechanisms by which Avastin fights cancer scientifically.

The Blood Vessel War

Avastin fights cancer in a unique way by concentrating on the blood arteries that support tumors rather than going after cancer cells directly. It is crucial to comprehend the critical role that angiogenesis—the development of new blood vessels—plays in the advancement of cancer in order to comprehend how Avastin functions.

The nutritional and oxygen requirements of cancer cells are very high. To continue growing, they need an efficient and steady flow of blood. Angiogenesis enters the picture here. Typically, a tumor emits chemicals that encourage the creation of new blood vessels from the preexisting vascular network, such as vascular endothelial growth factor (VEGF).

Avastin's Cunning Strategy

The main mechanism of action of avastin is inhibition of angiogenesis. The medication is made with VEGF, a crucial component that promotes the development of new blood vessels in tumors, as its specific target. Avastin efficiently inhibits the signals that cause angiogenesis by attaching to VEGF and blocking its interaction with receptors on blood vessel cells.

Consequently, the tumor loses its vital blood supply as the development of new blood vessels is impeded. This method effectively starves the tumor of oxygen and nourishment, much like cutting off its lifeline. The growth and spread of the tumor are greatly inhibited in the absence of a strong blood supply.

A Double-Beveled Blade

The anti-angiogenic properties of avastin affect cancer in two ways. First of all, by preventing the tumor from getting the resources it need to grow, it directly prevents tumor growth. This may result in the tumors that are already present shrinking in size and delaying their growth.

Second, and maybe just as significant, is that Avastin inhibits the growth of new metastases. Cancer is often particularly fatal because of metastasis, or the disease's ability to spread to other parts of the body. Avastin assists in preventing the tumor from dispersing "seeds" to form new colonies in other organs by inhibiting the angiogenesis process.

Improving Conventional Therapies

Chemotherapy and other conventional cancer treatments are frequently combined with avastin. The anti-angiogenic effect of the medication is leveraged in this combination method to enhance the delivery of chemotherapeutic drugs to the tumor. Avastin improves chemotherapy efficacy by regulating the tumor's blood arteries and decreasing their aberrant leakiness.

Avastin and chemotherapy together provide a multifaceted approach to combating cancer. Chemotherapy targets the cancer cells directly, boosting the chance of therapeutic success, while Avastin restricts the tumor's access to oxygen and nutrition.

A Targeted and Hopeful Method

The mode of action of Avastin demonstrates the promise of precision medicine in the management of cancer. By focusing on a particular biochemical pathway that is essential to the tumor's existence and growth, it lessens the harm that is done to healthy cells and lessens the side effects that are frequently connected to conventional treatments.

The activity of Avastin in clinical settings, its involvement in different types of cancer, and the inspiring true stories of patients who have benefited from its novel mechanism will all be covered in the chapters that follow. Avastin's strategy is not merely a window into the direction of cancer treatment; rather, it is evidence of the revolutionary force of science and technology in the continuous fight against cancer.

describing the mechanisms by which Avastin fights cancer scientifically.

The Blood Vessel War

Avastin employs a novel strategy in the fight against cancer. Instead of going straight after cancer cells, it goes after angiogenesis, a basic mechanism essential to the development and spread of cancers. Understanding the pivotal role angiogenesis plays in cancer is crucial to comprehending how Avastin functions.

Cancer cells devour oxygen and nutrients at a rapid rate. They need a steady and effective blood supply to sustain their unchecked and rapid growth. Angiogenesis enters the picture here. Typically, a tumor releases signaling chemicals to promote the creation of new blood vessels from the current network. One such molecule is vascular endothelial growth factor (VEGF).

Avastin's Cunning Strategy

The suppression of angiogenesis is crucial to the mechanism of action of avastin. The medication is specifically made to target VEGF, a vital component that promotes the growth of new blood vessels in tumors. Avastin effectively muffles the signals that trigger angiogenesis by binding to VEGF and preventing it from interacting with receptors on blood vessel cells.

The tumor loses its essential blood supply as a result of the inhibition of new blood vessel creation. This strategy is comparable to severing the tumor's oxygen and nutrition supply, so starving it to death. The growth and spread of the tumor are greatly inhibited in the absence of a strong blood supply.

A Double-Beveled Blade

The anti-angiogenic effect of avastin has two effects on cancer. First off, by preventing the tumor from getting the resources it needs to grow, it directly inhibits its growth. This frequently causes tumors that already exist to shrink, which slows the tumors' growth.

Secondly, and maybe just as importantly, Avastin inhibits the growth of new metastases. One of the main things that makes cancer especially deadly is metastasis, or the spread of the disease to other parts of the body. Avastin aids in preventing the tumor's ability to spread "seeds" to form new colonies in other organs by preventing angiogenesis.

Improving Conventional Therapies

Conventional cancer treatments like chemotherapy are frequently combined with avastin. This combined strategy makes use of Avastin's anti-angiogenic properties, which can improve the way chemotherapy drugs are delivered to the tumor. Avastin complements chemotherapy by regulating the tumor's blood arteries and reducing their aberrant permeability.

Chemotherapy and Avastin together constitute a multifaceted attack against cancer. Chemotherapy targets the cancer cells directly, whereas Avastin inhibits the tumor's ability to obtain oxygen and nutrition. The chance that treatment will be successful is increased by this dual attack.

A Targeted and Hopeful Method

The way that Avastin works is evidence of the promise that precision medicine has for treating cancer. By identifying a particular molecular route that is essential to the tumor's survival and growth, it reduces harm to healthy cells and lessens the adverse effects that are frequently connected to conventional therapies.

We will explore Avastin's activity in clinical settings, its significance in different types of cancer, and the inspiring true stories of patients who have benefited from its novel mechanism in further detail in the chapters that follow. Beyond offering a view into the future of cancer therapy, Avastin's method is a powerful example of how science and innovation may improve the ongoing fight against cancer.

Chapter 6: The Initial Cases of Success

testimonies from actual patients whose use of Avastin altered their lives.

Rebecca's Fortitude

Rebecca has experienced a turbulent road due to her disease. Her options appeared restricted after receiving a metastatic colorectal cancer diagnosis. She had gone through chemotherapy, surgeries, and the psychological rollercoaster of remission and recurrence. Rebecca's oncologist first gave her the medication Avastin during this battle.

Rebecca observed a shift soon after beginning Avastin. Her general well-being appeared to be improving, and her energy levels increased. The tumor's growth had stopped, according to scans, and her physician was cautiously optimistic. Rebecca saw Avastin as a glimmer of hope, giving her the opportunity to carry on making priceless memories with her family.

John's Courageous Journey

Glioblastoma multiforme is a severe form of brain cancer that John had to contend with. He and his loved ones were devastated by the diagnosis, but they did not waver in their resolve to look into every possible therapy option. Avastin became known as a possible saving grace.

Avastin's introduction into John's treatment plan was a game-changer. His recurring tumors, which had previously been inexorably growing, started to stabilize. The constant migraines and seizures that had turned into a daily struggle decreased in both frequency and severity. John's fight against glioblastoma was entering a stunning new chapter thanks to his tenacity and Avastin's assistance.

Emma's Victory Against Breast Cancer

Emma received a diagnosis of triple-negative breast cancer, which was as frightening as it was unpleasant. Avastin was added to the chemotherapy regimen as she started her treatment to increase her chances of recovery.

Emma had a life-changing encounter with Avastin. It not only shrank her tumor, but it also lessened the negative effects of her chemotherapy and made it easier to administer. Emma's cancer was defeated by the mix of treatments, which formed a strong coalition. Her experience was a striking example of how Avastin might help people who are receiving difficult cancer treatments live better lives.

An Upcoming Phase in the Battle Against Cancer

The influence that Avastin had in its early years is attested to by the accounts of Rebecca, John, Emma, and countless others. The medication was more than just a means of treatment; it stood for perseverance, optimism, and a new phase in the continuous battle against cancer.

With its distinct mode of action, avastin provided patients who had run out of choices for traditional treatment with a lifeline. It increased longevity, enhanced quality of life, and, in certain cases, offered a possibility of remission.

Patients' and healthcare professionals' aspirations were stoked by these true success tales. Avastin was more than just a medical breakthrough; it was a symbol of development, a confirmation that novel approaches to cancer treatment were not only feasible but also actively enhancing the quality of life for those coping with the severe obstacles associated with the disease.

We shall continue to examine Avastin's uses in various cancer types and how they affect patient outcomes in the ensuing chapters. These inspiring tales of tenacity and success highlight the game-changing potential of Avastin in the field of cancer treatment as well as the significant impact it has on the lives of individuals it affects.

CHAPTER 6

The First Success Stories

Real-life accounts of patients whose lives were changed by Avastin.

Rebecca's Fortitude

Rebecca's fight against cancer has been unrelenting. After receiving a diagnosis of metastatic colorectal cancer, she was thrust into an arduous journey involving numerous surgeries, chemotherapy, and the unpredictability of remission and relapse. Rebecca was first exposed to Avastin by her oncologist during this difficult time.

Avastin changed Rebecca's life in a way that was nothing short of miraculous. Her energy levels and general well-being significantly improved as soon as she started taking Avastin. The scans revealed a promising development: the tumor's growth had stopped. Her oncologist, who is often quiet about these things, started to sound cautiously optimistic. Avastin turned into a beacon of hope for Rebecca and her family as a whole. It gave her the opportunity to carry on leaving a legacy for her loved ones and capturing priceless moments.

John's Courageous Journey

Glioblastoma multiforme was a distressing diagnosis for John. Together with his loved ones, he faced an overwhelming task as a result of this extremely aggressive kind of brain cancer. Avastin appeared in the midst of the uncertainties as a glimmer of possible hope.

Avastin's addition to John's treatment plan was nothing short of revolutionary. The tumors that kept coming back, which had previously progressed without stopping, started to show indications of stabilization. The crippling headaches and seizures that had turned into a daily struggle started to lessen in frequency and severity. Together with John's bravery and tenacity, Avastin was writing a stunning new chapter in his fight against glioblastoma.

Emma's Victory Against Breast Cancer

When Emma received the news that she had triple-negative breast cancer, she faced an intimidating opponent. Avastin was added to chemotherapy as a crucial part of her treatment plan as she started her journey toward recovery in an effort to increase her chances of success.

Avastin turned become an invaluable ally for Emma. It not only helped shrink the size of her tumor, but it also made her chemotherapy program much easier to handle by minimizing the negative effects. Together, these treatments formed a powerful team that fought Emma's disease and ultimately helped her overcome her diagnosis.

An Upcoming Phase in the Battle Against Cancer

The testimonies of Rebecca, John, Emma, and several others who encountered the life-changing effects of Avastin signify not just personal triumphs but also noteworthy turning points in the battle against cancer. Avastin evolved into more than just a medication; it symbolized resiliency and optimism, and it signaled the start of a new phase in the continuous fight against cancer.

Avastin was providing patients who had run out of choices for conventional treatment with a lifeline thanks to its distinct mode of action. It was improving quality of life, extending life, and, in certain cases, providing hope for remission. These true success stories had a significant influence on medical professionals, researchers, patients, and their families.

These tales acted as potent reminders that advancements in cancer treatment and medical innovation were actively improving the lives of people dealing with the severe obstacles posed by cancer, not just theoretically. With the development of Avastin, a new chapter in the history of cancer treatment began, one that promises patients meaningful outcomes and is defined by optimism and resiliency.

We will continue to examine Avastin's wide range of uses in different cancer types and its growing influence on patient outcomes in the upcoming chapters. These inspiring tales of tenacity and success offer strong proof of Avastin's revolutionary potential in the field of cancer treatment as well as its significant impact on the lives of people it affects.

CHAPTER 7

The Battle Against Resistance
Addressing challenges and setbacks in using Avastin for cancer treatment.

The Intricacy of Cancer

Avastin has been a ray of hope for cancer patients, but the road has not been without difficulties. A powerful enemy is cancer's intricacy and capacity for adaptation and evolution. Certain cancer cells may become resistant to medications, such as Avastin, over time.

Avastin resistance can develop via a variety of methods. Avastin targets the VEGF pathway, and one typical process is the development of mutations in this pathway. Because the tumor can continue to grow despite the presence of Avastin due to these modifications, the medication may become less effective.

The Microenvironment's Function

The tumor microenvironment is another factor to take into account. Cancer cells have the ability to change their environment in order to stimulate angiogenesis and evade the effects of Avastin. This may involve the production of different pro-angiogenic signals or the recruitment of immune cells that stimulate the formation of blood vessels. Such flexibility can make treatment plans more difficult to implement and present obstacles in the fight against cancer.

Overcoming Opposition

One of the difficult aspects of utilizing Avastin to treat cancer is the development of resistance. When dealing with resistance, a multifaceted strategy is frequently used. Scholars and medical professionals are consistently exploring novel approaches to augment the efficacy of Avastin and postpone or surmount resistance.

Creating combination treatments that address several facets of the tumor microenvironment is one strategy. Combinations such as Avastin with other immunotherapies or targeted therapies are possible; these treatments cooperate to obstruct resistance processes.

Finding biomarkers that can indicate which patients are more likely to respond to Avastin and which are more likely to develop resistance is another area of active research. Treatment regimens that are tailored to each patient's specific tumor biology are becoming more and more crucial.

The Battle That Never Stops

The struggle against resistance is an ever-changing and continuous one. Novel approaches to combating resistance will surface as our comprehension of the mechanisms behind both cancer and Avastin continues to grow. It's critical to understand that, despite these difficulties, Avastin is still an indispensable weapon in the fight against cancer, providing increased survival, enhanced quality of life, and the possibility of significant results.

We will examine how Avastin is used in contemporary cancer treatment, the research being done to overcome resistance, and the experiences of patients who continue to benefit from this novel treatment in the chapters that follow. The fight against resistance is evidence of the medical community's tenacity and persistent commitment to giving patients the best chance possible in their battle with cancer.

discussing the difficulties and failures associated with treating cancer using Avastin.

The Intricacy of Cancer

The complexity of cancer presents a significant obstacle in the fight against the illness. Avastin has been a ray of optimism, but there have been challenges along the way. Cancer is a dynamic foe that is renowned for its capacity for change and adaptation. Certain cancer cells may become resistant to medications, such as Avastin, over time.

Avastin resistance can appear via a number of different methods. Avastin targets the VEGF pathway, and one typical mechanism is the development of mutations in this pathway. Because the tumor can continue to grow despite the presence of Avastin due to these modifications, the medication may become less effective.

The Tumor Microenvironment's Function

The formation of resistance is significantly influenced by the tumor microenvironment. Cancer cells have the ability to change their environment in order to stimulate angiogenesis and evade the effects of Avastin. This manipulation may entail the production of alternate pro-angiogenic signals or the recruitment of immune cells that stimulate the formation of blood vessels. These modifications may make treatment plans more difficult to implement and provide serious obstacles in the continuous fight against cancer.

Overcoming Opposition

Dealing with resistance is a difficult task that frequently calls for a multifaceted strategy. Scholars and medical professionals are consistently exploring novel approaches to augment the efficacy of Avastin and postpone or surmount resistance.

Creating combo therapy is one important strategy. Avastin may be used in conjunction with other immunotherapies or targeted treatments in these combinations. By addressing many facets of the tumor microenvironment, these combination treatments aim to prevent the emergence of resistance. Together, these treatments have a synergistic effect that frequently delays or eliminates the adaptive processes used by cancer cells.

Moreover, current studies focus on finding biomarkers that can indicate which patients are more likely to respond to Avastin and which are more likely to have resistance. Making the best treatment decisions increasingly depends on customized therapy regimens that take into account each patient's particular tumor biology.

The Battle That Never Stops

The struggle against resistance is a constant state of flux. New methods of combating resistance will keep arriving as our comprehension of the mechanisms behind both cancer and Avastin deepens. It is critical to understand that avastin is still an important weapon in the fight against cancer, despite the difficulties. Patients may have a longer chance of survival, a higher quality of life, and the potential for significant results.

The use of Avastin in contemporary cancer treatment, current research to overcome resistance, and patient success stories with this novel medicine will all be covered in the chapters that follow. The medical community's tenacity and persistent commitment to giving patients the best opportunity possible in their fight against cancer are demonstrated by the battle against resistance. Even if there are many obstacles to overcome, there are also many innovations that are changing the face of cancer treatment.

CHAPTER 8

Expanding the Reach: Avastin in Different Cancers Discussing the diverse applications of Avastin in various cancer types.

talking about the many uses of Avastin for different kinds of cancer.

Hepatocellular Cancer

Metastatic colorectal cancer was the first malignancy for which Avastin was used as a treatment. It has a significant impact on this field. Avastin significantly increased overall survival as well as progression-free survival when combined with chemotherapy. It gave patients a longer life expectancy and the ability to better manage their illness, and it soon became the norm for medical care.

Chest Cancer

Avastin's launch was seen as a potential game-changer for non-small cell lung cancer, a condition that is known for being extremely difficult to treat. For non-squamous non-small cell lung cancer, as part of first-line therapy, avastin has received approval. It was an essential adjunct to chemotherapy that changed the course of lung cancer treatment and increased overall survival.

Maternal Cancer

Avastin has provided a glimpse of hope in the field of breast cancer, namely in the aggressive triple-negative subtype. It worked well in conjunction with chemotherapy to shrink tumors and increase the likelihood of a successful surgical excision. Avastin has encountered difficulties along the way, but it is still an important weapon in the fight against breast cancer.

Multiple Glioblastoma Types

Avastin had outstanding results in the treatment of glioblastoma multiforme, an extremely aggressive brain cancer. It provided a longer progression-free survival as well as improved quality of life for patients facing this powerful foe. Avastin came to represent advancement in an area with few available treatments.

Breast Cancer

Avastin also showed promise for treating ovarian cancer, which is frequently detected at an advanced stage. When paired with chemotherapy, Avastin demonstrated its capacity to stall the advancement of the disease, providing patients with additional time and optimism to combat this difficult malignancy.

An Integrated Method

The promise and versatility of Avastin are demonstrated by its many applications in different forms of cancer. It emphasizes how crucial precision medicine is to the treatment of cancer, as treatments are customized to the unique features of each patient's malignancy.

Avastin's journey has not been without difficulties and disappointments, but there is no denying that it has had a profound effect on the area of cancer therapy. It has increased the range of possible treatments, providing patients with additional choices, increasing their chances of survival, and improving their quality of life while undergoing therapy.

We will continue to examine Avastin's uses in various cancer types, continuing research aimed at extending its therapeutic range, and patient success stories illustrating its novel approach in the upcoming chapters. The discovery that astantin is present in several tumors is a major advancement in the ongoing battle against these difficult and complex illnesses.

talking about the many uses of Avastin for different kinds of cancer.

Hepatocellular Cancer

The first application of avastin in the treatment of metastatic colorectal cancer occurred in this context. It had a very revolutionary effect on this specific sort of cancer. Avastin significantly increased patients' overall survival and progression-free survival when added to chemotherapy regimens. It quickly became the norm for treatment, giving patients with metastatic colorectal cancer not just a longer life expectancy but also a better chance of controlling their condition.

Chest Cancer

Another condition that is known to be extremely difficult to treat is non-small cell lung cancer, for which Avastin has emerged as a possible game-changer. Approved as an essential part of first-line treatment for non-small cell, non-squamous lung cancer, is Avastin. It changed the course of lung cancer treatment and improved overall survival rates when added to chemotherapy regimens. The use of avastin in the treatment of lung cancer demonstrates both its versatility in treating many cancer types and its potential to have a major effect in a range of therapeutic contexts.

Maternal Cancer

Avastin has given promise in the treatment of breast cancer, especially in the case of the aggressive triple-negative subtype. It has been shown to be useful in lowering tumor size and improving the likelihood of a successful surgical excision when combined with chemotherapy regimens. Avastin has faced obstacles along the way, but despite this, it is still a useful weapon in the complicated and varied fight against breast cancer.

Multiple Glioblastoma Types

Avastin had outstanding results in the treatment of glioblastoma multiforme, an extremely aggressive brain cancer. For patients facing this powerful enemy, it provided a longer progression-free survival and improved quality of life. In a profession with historically few treatment choices, Avastin came to represent advancement. Its effect on glioblastoma multiforme highlighted precision medicine's potential in the fight for more effective treatment alternatives.

Breast Cancer

Avastin also showed promise for treating ovarian cancer, which is frequently detected at an advanced stage. Avastin demonstrated its ability to slow the course of the disease when administered in conjunction with chemotherapy, giving patients additional time and hope to fight this difficult malignancy. The use of Avastin in the treatment of ovarian cancer demonstrated how it can expand the application of cutting-edge treatments to a range of clinical settings.

An Integrated Method

The potential and versatility of Avastin are highlighted by its many applications in different forms of cancer. This highlights the value of precision medicine in the treatment of cancer, as treatments are tailored to the particulars of each patient's malignancy. Because of its versatility, Avastin has demonstrated that it is not just a medication for a single form of cancer but rather an all-purpose instrument in the oncologist's toolbox.

Despite some difficulties along the way, Avastin has unquestionably had a profound effect on the area of cancer therapy. It has increased the range of possible treatments, providing patients with additional choices, increasing their chances of survival, and improving their quality of life while undergoing therapy.

We will continue to examine Avastin's uses in various cancer types, continuing research aimed at extending its therapeutic range, and patient success stories illustrating its novel approach in the upcoming chapters. The discovery that asvastin is found in several malignancies is a major advancement in the ongoing fight against these difficult and complex illnesses, providing hope to individuals who are battling cancer.

CHAPTER 9

The Controversies Surrounding Avastin
Examining the debates and controversies related to Avastin's efficacy and side effects.

analyzing the arguments and disputes surrounding the effectiveness and negative effects of Avastin.

Assistiveness for Breast Cancer

The use of Avastin in the treatment of breast cancer has been one of the main topics of contention. Even though the medication was approved and showed early promise, further clinical research cast doubt on its efficacy. Studies that did not demonstrate a statistically significant increase in overall survival gave rise to discussions over whether the possible advantages exceeded the expenses and hazards.

2011 saw the U.S. The FDA withdrew its approval of Avastin as a therapy for breast cancer. This choice caused a stir in the community, with some arguing that the medication should still be available because certain people could still benefit from it.

Adverse Reactions

The adverse effects of Avastin have generated discussion. Despite the medication's specific mode of action, it may also have an impact on healthy blood vessels, which could result in adverse effects like bleeding, hypertension, or gastrointestinal perforations. It has proven to be a difficult effort for patients and healthcare providers to weigh these negative effects against the possible advantages of treatment.

Expense and Availability

Another point of contention has been Avastin's exorbitant price. Many people may find it too expensive to obtain, and there have been ongoing discussions about the drug's cost-effectiveness. Avastin pricing and accessibility have been divisive topics, especially in nations without national healthcare programs.

Current Studies and Discussions

Clinical studies and ongoing research have not been hindered by the controversy surrounding Avastin. Scholars are still looking into possible uses for the medication and ways to make it more efficient. Debate continues to center on the relative merits of Avastin vs its adverse effects as well as the drug's role in the larger context of cancer treatment.

Views from Patients

The opinions of patients are also very important in the discussions around Avastin. Some people's cancer journeys have been saved by the medication since it has given them hope for a longer life and a higher quality of life. It's possible that some people had negative effects that offset any possible advantages. The need for individualized treatment options in cancer care is highlighted by the variety of patient experiences.

A Complicated Terrain

The disputes pertaining to Avastin serve as a prime example of the intricate terrain of cancer therapy. A complex task is striking a balance between cost, side effects, effectiveness, and patient preferences. The development of Avastin in the treatment of breast cancer and other areas has served as an example of the value of evidence-based decision-making and the continuous search for novel approaches in the fight against cancer.

We will explore Avastin's changing position in cancer treatment, its continued obstacles, and the true accounts of patients whose lives have been impacted by this ground-breaking medication in the ensuing chapters. The debates around Avastin provide guidance for moving forward in this always changing fight against a powerful foe by serving as a reminder of the difficulties and moral issues involved in cancer therapy.

analyzing the arguments and disputes surrounding the effectiveness and negative effects of Avastin.

Assistiveness for Breast Cancer

The use of Avastin in the treatment of breast cancer has been one of the main topics of contention. At first, it was approved by the authorities and showed a lot of potential. But as further clinical trials were carried out, doubts regarding the medication's general efficacy in this situation started to surface. Several trials did not show a statistically significant increase in overall survival, which cast question on whether the possible advantages outweighed the dangers and expenses involved.

2011 saw the U.S. The FDA made the decision to withdraw Avastin's approval as a treatment for breast cancer. This choice sparked a heated debate. Proponents contended that even though the medication may not be beneficial for all patients, access to it should be preserved because some people did show benefits from it.

Adverse Reactions

Debatable have been Avastin's negative effects as well. The medicine can also impact normal blood arteries, even though its mechanism of action is directed towards the blood vessels supplying malignancies. Side effects include bleeding, hypertension, or the extremely uncommon case of gastrointestinal tract perforations could result from this. For both patients and healthcare professionals, weighing these negative effects against the possible advantages of treatment has proven to be a difficult task.

Expense and Availability

Another major point of contention has been Avastin's high price. Many people may find it difficult to obtain the medication due to its cost, especially if they do not have full health insurance. Discussions about Avastin's cost-effectiveness have been going on for a while, and some stakeholders are worried about the financial strain it puts on healthcare systems.

Current Studies and Discussions

Avastin-related research and clinical studies are still being carried out in spite of the controversy. Researchers are looking into how the medication might be used to treat different kinds of cancer and are actively looking for ways to make it more successful. The relative advantages and disadvantages of Avastin, as well as its place in the larger scheme of cancer therapy alternatives, are still hotly contested issues.

Views from Patients

Debates pertaining to Avastin require the inclusion of patient perspectives. Avastin has given some people hope for a longer life expectancy and a higher standard of living. It has given them hope and significant results, acting as a lifeline throughout their cancer battle. However, some people have had adverse consequences that have overshadowed any possible advantages. The variety of patient experiences highlights the importance of individualised and patient-focused decision-making in cancer treatment.

A Complicated Terrain

The Avastin controversy serves as an example of the complex and multidimensional terrain of cancer treatment. It might be difficult to strike a balance between factors like patient preferences, side effects, cost, and effectiveness. The development of Avastin in the treatment of breast cancer and other areas emphasizes the value of evidence-based decision-making and the continuous search for novel approaches in the fight against cancer.

We will explore Avastin's changing position in cancer treatment, ongoing obstacles, and the true accounts of patients whose lives have been touched by this ground-breaking medication in the upcoming chapters. The debates around Avastin serve as a timely reminder of the difficulties and moral dilemmas associated with cancer treatment. They provide direction in the never-ending fight against a powerful foe, emphasizing the necessity of ongoing assessment and adjustment in the quest for improved cancer treatment.

CHAPTER 10

Beyond Medicine: Avastin's Impact on Patients' Lives Stories of how Avastin affected patients' quality of life and emotional well-being.

Accounts of the effects of Avastin on patients' emotional health and quality of life.

Emily's Newfound Vigor

Emily was emotionally and physically exhausted from her fight against metastatic colorectal cancer. Her treatment cycle had left her exhausted and demoralized. A change started to occur when her oncologist added Avastin to her treatment regimen. She seemed to come alive around Avastin. She felt more like herself again and had more energy. Not only did this rejuvenation benefit her physically, but it also greatly enhanced her emotional health. Her will to carry on the battle was fueled by the optimism and vigor that Avastin offered.

David's Passage of Typicality

David's life has completely changed after receiving a non-small cell lung cancer diagnosis. The illness has changed the course of his everyday life in addition to endangering his physical health. The addition of Avastin to his treatment plan was a game-changer. He was able to restore his sense of normalcy when his tumors started to react. Even though it was just temporary, having this feeling of control over his life had a profound effect on his emotional health. It restored happy times, get-togethers with loved ones, and treasured memories that lung cancer had momentarily taken away.

Sarah's Feeling of Independence

Sarah felt powerless after being diagnosed with triple-negative breast cancer. Her well-being was negatively impacted by the adverse effects of her treatment, which frequently left her vulnerable. She saw a change after adding Avastin to her treatment. It not only helped shrink the size of her tumor but also lessened the negative effects of her chemotherapy, making it easier to administer. Sarah's perspective was altered by her newly discovered sense of authority. Beyond the treatment's tangible effects, she felt as though she had taken back control of her life.

Tom's Prolonged Stay with His Family

Tom's time with his family had been jeopardized by glioblastoma multiforme. At first, the diagnosis seemed like a death sentence, but there was a ray of hope with Avastin. It improved his quality of life and prolonged his progression-free survival. For Tom, this meant having more quality time with his family, experiencing more moments together, and witnessing his kids develop. The immense emotional benefits that Avastin offered were peace of mind and the chance to keep creating memories with the people he cared about.

The Medical Field's Human Face

The human side of medicine is best illustrated by the tales of Emily, David, Sarah, Tom, and numerous others. Beyond the clinical metrics and data, Avastin has had a significant positive effect on patients' quality of life and emotional health in addition to survival rates.

These accounts highlight the comprehensive approach to cancer care, in which medications such as Avastin not only target tumors but also give patients newfound hope, courage, and fortitude to battle on. They stress that providing treatment for cancer patients involves more than just medicine and takes into account their emotional, psychological, and social needs.

We will continue to examine the complex effects of Avastin on patients' life, the continuous improvements in cancer treatment, and the changing field of cancer treatment in the upcoming chapters. The inspirational tales of human tenacity and optimism serve as a reminder that, in the face of cancer, medical innovation can transcend medicine and touch the very core of existence.

Accounts of the effects of Avastin on patients' emotional health and quality of life.

Emily's Newfound Vigor

Emily had faced several difficulties during her fight with metastatic colorectal cancer. She was exhausted from the constant chemotherapy's toll on her body and mind. However, it appeared as though a glimmer of hope had finally emerged when her physician included Avastin in her treatment regimen. Emily's life had a renewed sense of vibrancy and energy thanks to Avastin. She began to feel like an active participant in her life rather than just an observer. This renewal was not just physical but also had a significant effect on her mental health. Her drive to carry on the fight was fueled by the hope and energy that Avastin offered.

David's Passage of Typicality

David's life has completely changed after receiving a non-small cell lung cancer diagnosis. The illness had disturbed his daily routine in addition to endangering his physical well-being. An important turning point in his treatment was the addition of Avastin to his regimen. David saw that he was starting to feel a bit more normal as his tumors started to react to the medication. He could spend time with his loved ones, engage in activities he used to like, and feel somewhat in control of his life again. This sense of control represented a significant emotional shift in addition to a physical one. It was as though Avastin had restored to him the happy times, family get-togethers, and treasured memories that lung cancer had momentarily taken away.

Sarah's Feeling of Independence

Sarah's triple-negative breast cancer had sometimes made her feel powerless. Her well-being had been steadily eroded by the side effects of her treatment, which frequently felt like a rollercoaster. Avastin's introduction into her treatment plan was a substantial change. It not only helped shrink the size of her tumor but also lessened the negative effects of her chemotherapy, making it easier to administer. Sarah was cognizant of her recently discovered sense of authority. Beyond the treatment's tangible effects, she felt as though she had taken back control of her life. She was able to confront the difficulties posed by cancer with more optimism and fortitude thanks to her emotional resilience.

Tom's Prolonged Stay with His Family

A glioblastoma multiforme diagnosis had felt like the end of the world for Tom. He had lived a long life under the cloud of uncertainty surrounding his diagnosis. Avastin, though, offered some optimism. It improved his quality of life and prolonged his progression-free survival. More time with his family was an incalculable benefit for Tom as a result. It meant more time spent together, more giggles, and the chance to see his kids grow up. One significant benefit of Avastin was emotional well-being. It allowed him to continue creating memories with the people he loved and brought him a sense of serenity. His fight against cancer evolved into an emotional triumph rather than merely a medical one.

The Medical Field's Human Face

The human side of medicine is best illustrated by the tales of Emily, David, Sarah, Tom, and numerous others. Avastin has had a significant influence on patients' lives that goes beyond clinical measurements and statistics. It's about improving life quality and emotional stability, not only about prolonging survival.

These accounts highlight the comprehensive approach to cancer care, in which medications such as Avastin not only target tumors but also give patients newfound hope, courage, and fortitude to battle on. They stress that providing treatment for cancer patients involves more than just medicine and takes into account their emotional, psychological, and social needs.

We will continue to examine the complex effects of Avastin on patients' life, the continuous improvements in cancer treatment, and the changing field of cancer treatment in the upcoming chapters. The inspirational tales of human tenacity and optimism serve as a reminder that, in the face of cancer, medical innovation can transcend medicine and touch the very core of existence. These tales demonstrate the enormous influence that cutting-edge cancer treatments may have on patients' emotional and psychological fortitude in the face of hardship in addition to their physical health.

CHAPTER 11

Navigating the Challenges of Avastin Treatment Providing guidance on managing side effects and treatment-related difficulties.

provide direction on how to handle side effects and challenges arising from treatment.

Handling Adverse Reactions

Like all cancer treatments, avastin medication might have adverse effects that need to be carefully managed. For patients to overcome these obstacles, strong collaboration between them and their healthcare providers is necessary. Here's a closer look at how to handle typical Avastin side effects:

Blood Pressure Control: In certain people, avastin may cause an increase in blood pressure. It is essential to regularly check blood pressure before, during, and after treatment. It is possible to administer medication to treat hypertension. Under the supervision of a healthcare professional, patients should also- adopt a heart-healthy lifestyle, which includes a low-sodium diet and frequent exercise.

Precautions Against Bleeding: Patients should be made aware of the warning signs of bleeding, which include easy bruising, nosebleeds, and blood in the stool or urine. Non-steroidal anti-inflammatory drug (NSAID) use must be avoided, and any bleeding concerns should be discussed as soon as possible with healthcare experts.

Monitoring for Proteinuria: Avastin may cause proteinuria, or an overabundance of protein in the urine. Frequent urine testing can assist in early proteinuria detection. Patients should notify their healthcare staff of any changes in the color or frequency of their urine, since this may require modifications to their treatment plan.

Gastrointestinal Health: Patients should exercise caution and report any symptoms of nausea, vomiting, or abdominal discomfort as soon as they occur, even though Avastin seldom causes direct gastrointestinal side effects. Lowering the risk of gastrointestinal perforations can be achieved by abstaining from aspirin and NSAID use.

Emotional Assistance

It can be emotionally taxing to deal with cancer and its treatment, especially Avastin. During this process, getting emotional support is essential. Here's how to handle the sentimental parts:

Support Groups: Becoming a member of a cancer support group can give you a sense of belonging and empathy. It can be incredibly consoling to share worries and experiences with people who are traveling a similar journey.

Psychological Counseling: When navigating the emotional challenges of a cancer diagnosis and treatment, patients and their loved ones might benefit from professional counseling or therapy. Strategies for managing stress, anxiety, and depression can be obtained by speaking with a mental health expert.

Friends and Family: Rely on your network of friends and family for support. You can share your worries and get the emotional support you require by having open and honest conversations with others. Don't be afraid to ask for help; loved ones typically wish to assist.

Self-Care: It's essential to look after your mental and emotional health. Take up hobbies, relaxation techniques, or peaceful, joyful pursuits. Continuing this self-care is crucial to preserving emotional toughness.

Consumption and Activity

Exercise and good nutrition are essential for maintaining a patient's general health and resilience to the side effects of Avastin treatment. Here are some thorough pointers:

Balanced Diet: Work with a trained dietitian to create a diet that is both balanced and meets your unique nutritional requirements while undergoing treatment. They can offer advice on how to handle dietary difficulties like appetite loss, taste alterations, and digestive problems.

Physical Activity: Make sure you get regular exercise, but make sure you follow your doctor's instructions. Exercise can enhance your general well-being, help you feel more energised, and manage treatment-related weariness.

Hydration: It's critical to maintain enough hydration, particularly if you have adverse effects like proteinuria. Constipation is one of the side effects of cancer treatment that can be managed with an adequate fluid intake.

Rest: The body needs enough sleep and rest to rebuild and mend. Getting enough sleep is essential to controlling fatigue, a common side effect of cancer treatment.

Interaction with Medical Professionals

Throughout your Avastin therapy, it is imperative that you maintain open and honest communication with your healthcare team. Please do not hesitate to contact your healthcare practitioner if you have any questions, concerns, or adverse effects. They can make changes to your treatment regimen, suggest new resources, or offer strategies to better control side effects.

A thorough, multidisciplinary strategy that takes into account the practical, emotional, and physical components of the patient's journey is necessary to navigate the hurdles of Avastin treatment. Patients are able to effectively manage side effects and treatment-related issues if they are provided with appropriate techniques, support, and communication. This promotes their general well-being and resilience against cancer, in addition to improving their quality of life during treatment.

Handling Adverse Reactions

Like all cancer treatments, avastin medication might have adverse effects that need to be carefully managed. To successfully negotiate these obstacles, strong collaboration between patients and their healthcare providers is necessary. Here's a closer look at how to handle typical Avastin side effects:

Blood Pressure Management: In certain people, avastin may cause an increase in blood pressure. It is essential to regularly check blood pressure before, during, and after treatment. It is possible to administer medication to treat hypertension. Under the supervision of a healthcare professional, patients should also adopt a heart-healthy lifestyle that includes a low-sodium diet, frequent exercise, and stress-reduction practices.

Precautions Against Bleeding: Patients should be made aware of the warning signs of bleeding, which include easy bruising, nosebleeds, and blood in the stool or urine. Non-steroidal anti-inflammatory medicines (NSAIDs) must never be used, and any bleeding concerns should be promptly addressed with a healthcare physician. If bleeding happens, the medical staff can evaluate how serious it is and decide on the best course of action.

Monitoring for Proteinuria: Avastin may cause proteinuria, or an overabundance of protein in the urine. Frequent urine testing can assist in early proteinuria detection. Patients should notify their healthcare staff of any changes in the color, frequency, or appearance of foamy urine. Dietary changes and medicines may be necessary to manage proteinuria and preserve renal function.

Gastrointestinal Health: Patients should exercise caution and report any symptoms of nausea, vomiting, or abdominal discomfort as soon as they occur, even though Avastin seldom causes direct gastrointestinal side effects. Lowering the risk of gastrointestinal perforations can be achieved by abstaining from aspirin and NSAID use. To support their gastrointestinal health, patients should eat a mild, balanced diet. If they have any concerns, they should speak with their healthcare practitioners.

Emotional Assistance

It can be emotionally taxing to deal with cancer and its treatment, especially Avastin. During this process, getting emotional support is essential. Here's how to handle the sentimental parts:

Support Groups: Becoming a member of a cancer support group can give you a sense of belonging and empathy. It can be incredibly consoling to share worries and experiences with people who are traveling a similar journey. These gathering places frequently offer a forum for talking about emotional difficulties and exchanging coping mechanisms.

Psychological Counseling: When navigating the emotional challenges of a cancer diagnosis and treatment, patients and their loved ones might benefit from professional counseling or therapy. Speaking with a mental health professional can offer coping mechanisms for managing stress, anxiety, and depression as well as a secure setting for discussing and resolving emotional difficulties.

Friends and Family: Rely on your network of friends and family for support. You can share your worries and get the emotional support you require by having open and honest conversations with others. Don't be afraid to ask for help when you need it—your loved ones are usually willing to lend a hand.

Self-Care: It's essential to look after your mental and emotional health. Take up hobbies, relaxation techniques, or peaceful, joyful pursuits. Taking care of yourself is essential when coping with cancer, not a luxury. It supports the preservation of emotional fortitude and self-control.

Consumption and Activity

Exercise and good nutrition are essential for maintaining a patient's general health and resilience to the side effects of Avastin treatment. Here are some thorough pointers:

Balanced Diet: Work with a trained dietitian to create a diet that is both balanced and meets your unique nutritional requirements while undergoing treatment. They can offer advice on how to handle dietary difficulties like appetite loss, taste alterations, and digestive problems. Eating a range of meals high in nutrients, such as whole grains, fruits, vegetables, and lean proteins, can improve your general health.

Physical Activity: Make sure you get regular exercise, but make sure you follow your doctor's instructions. Exercise can enhance your general well-being, help you feel more energised, and manage treatment-related weariness. Even simple activity can have a big impact, like walking or even yoga.

Hydration: It's critical to maintain enough hydration, particularly if you have adverse effects like proteinuria. Constipation is one of the side effects of cancer treatment that can be managed with an adequate fluid intake. Regular use of water and other hydrating beverages is advised throughout the day.

Rest: The body needs enough sleep and rest to rebuild and mend. Getting enough sleep is essential to controlling fatigue, a common side effect of cancer treatment. To get better quality sleep, set up a regular sleep pattern, make your sleeping space cozy, and engage in relaxation exercises.

Interaction with Medical Professionals

Throughout your Avastin therapy, it is imperative that you maintain open and honest communication with your healthcare team. Please do not hesitate to contact your healthcare practitioner if you have any questions, concerns, or adverse effects. They can make changes to your treatment regimen, suggest new resources, or offer strategies to better control side effects. Your well-being is the first priority of your healthcare team, who are there to assist you in overcoming the obstacles of therapy.

A thorough, multidisciplinary strategy that takes into account the practical, emotional, and physical components of the patient's journey is necessary to navigate the hurdles of Avastin treatment. Patients are able to effectively manage side effects and treatment-related issues if they are provided with appropriate techniques, support, and communication. This promotes their general well-being and resilience against cancer, in addition to improving their quality of life during treatment. Although the path may be difficult, it is one that can be traveled with hope and strength if the correct help and direction are provided.

Chapter 11: Handling the Difficulties of Avastin Therapy

provide direction on how to handle side effects and challenges arising from treatment.

Handling Adverse Reactions

Side effects from avastin medication can occur, so it's critical that patients and medical professionals collaborate to handle these issues.

Avastin frequently causes hypertension, or high blood pressure, bleeding, proteinuria, or an excess of protein in the urine, and gastrointestinal perforations. The following tactics can be used to manage these negative effects:

Blood Pressure Management: It's critical to regularly check your blood pressure. It is possible to administer medications to treat hypertension. Patients are frequently encouraged to lead heart-healthy lifestyles, which include frequent exercise and a low-sodium diet.

Precautions Against Bleeding: Patients need to be informed about the warning signs of bleeding, which include easy bruising, nosebleeds, and blood in the stool or urine. It's critical to refrain from using non-steroidal anti-inflammatory medicines (NSAIDs) and to see a doctor if you have any worries about bleeding.

Monitoring for Proteinuria: Frequent urine testing can assist in early detection of proteinuria. Notifying your healthcare staff of any changes in the color or frequency of your urine is very important.

Gastrointestinal Health: Patients should exercise caution and report right once any symptoms of nausea, vomiting, or stomach pain. The risk of gastrointestinal perforations can be decreased by abstaining from aspirin and NSAIDs.

Emotional Assistance

Emotional health can be negatively impacted by coping with cancer and its treatments, such as

Avastin. During this process, getting emotional support is crucial. Here are some strategies for overcoming the emotional obstacles:

Support Groups: Becoming a member of a cancer support group can give you a sense of belonging and empathy. It can be incredibly consoling to share worries and experiences with people who are traveling a similar route.

Psychological Counseling: When navigating the emotional challenges of a cancer diagnosis and treatment, patients and their loved ones might benefit from professional counseling or therapy.

Friends and Family: Rely on your network of friends and family for support. You can share your worries and get the emotional support you require by having open and honest conversations with others.

Self-Care: It's essential to look after your mental and emotional health. Take up hobbies, relaxation techniques, or peaceful, joyful pursuits.

Consumption and Activity

Patients may be better able to handle the difficulties of Avastin treatment if they continue to follow a balanced diet and lifestyle. The following advice relates to exercise and nutrition:

Balanced Diet: During therapy, create a balanced diet that suits your individual needs by working with a trained dietitian.

Physical Activity: As directed by your healthcare professional, get regular exercise. Engaging in physical activity can enhance your vitality and general health.

Hydration: It's critical to maintain enough hydration, particularly if you have adverse effects like proteinuria.

Rest: The body needs enough sleep and rest to rebuild and mend.

Interaction with Medical Professionals

It's critical that you and your healthcare team communicate openly and clearly during your Avastin treatment. Do not hesitate to contact your healthcare practitioner if you have questions or encounter side effects. They can suggest more help or modify your treatment strategy.

A multidisciplinary strategy that takes into account the patient's physical, emotional, and practical needs is necessary to navigate the hurdles of Avastin treatment. Patients can successfully manage side effects and treatment-related issues with the correct techniques and assistance, which will ultimately improve their quality of life while undergoing treatment.

CHAPTER 12

The Future of Cancer Treatment Discussing the role of Avastin in shaping the future of oncology.

First of all,

Cancer treatment has advanced significantly, and oncology appears to have a bright future thanks to advances in medical science. One important factor influencing how cancer is treated in the future is Avastin (bevacizumab), a novel medication that has completely changed the oncology industry. The function of Avastin in cancer treatment and its possible effects on cancer care in the future are examined in this chapter.

Recognizing Avastin:

Vascular endothelial growth factor (VEGF) is the target of the monoclonal antibody Avastin. Angiogenesis, the process by which new blood vessels grow, is greatly aided by this protein. Angiogenesis is a crucial component of cancer that permits tumors to proliferate and spread. By blocking VEGF, avastin prevents the growth of new blood vessels inside the tumor, thereby depriving it of the oxygen and nutrition it needs to survive.

Avastin in Treatment for Cancer:

Colorectal Cancer: When Avastin was first licensed in 2004 for the treatment of metastatic colorectal cancer, it brought about a dramatic change in the way that cancer is treated. As one of the first medications to specifically target angiogenesis, it gave patients with advanced colorectal cancer new hope.

Growing Usage: As time has gone on, Avastin's uses have expanded to include kidney, lung, and breast cancers, among other cancer types. Because of its capacity to impede angiogenesis, it is a useful ingredient in many combination treatments.

Increasing Survival Rates: Numerous cancer patients' progression-free survival has been demonstrated to be improved by avastin. Better overall survival rates have resulted from this, which is a noteworthy advancement in cancer care.

Difficulties and Debates:

Despite being heralded as a revolutionary treatment in oncology, Avastin has not been without controversy. Among the difficulties and worries pertaining to its use are:

Avastin side effects include bleeding, gastrointestinal perforations, and elevated blood pressure. For patient safety, controlling these adverse effects is essential.

High Costs: Many patients may not be able to afford or obtain Avastin or other targeted medicines due to their high cost.

Prospective Routes:

The therapy of cancer has a bright future ahead of it, and Avastin will probably be a key player in determining that future. Avastin is anticipated to have a lasting effect in the following important areas:

Combination Therapies: To increase Avastin's efficacy and lessen its negative effects, researchers are investigating the drug's potential when combined with other medications.

Precision Medicine: The identification of people most likely to benefit from Avastin's therapeutic potential will likely be made possible by developments in genomics and customized medicine.

Ongoing study: New understandings of the mechanisms and uses of Avastin will be uncovered via ongoing study, opening the door to even more developments in the fight against cancer.

In summary:

By focusing on angiogenesis, a key mechanism in the development of cancer, Avastin has made a substantial contribution to the treatment of cancer in the future. Its influence on the development of the oncology landscape is significant, despite the difficulties and disagreements that it faces. Avastin's role in the fight against cancer is still significant as research and treatment advances, providing patients with hope and a bright future for the field of oncology.

Of course, let's examine in more detail how Avastin will influence oncology going forward:

Progress in Combination Treatments:

Avastin's potential for use in combination therapy is one of the interesting aspects of its function in cancer treatment going forward. The goal of continuing research is to find synergistic medicine combinations that maximize benefits and minimize drawbacks from Avastin. Combination therapy is this strategy, and it has already demonstrated promise in treating a variety of cancer types.

For instance, Avastin is frequently used in conjunction with chemotherapy drugs like paclitaxel to treat lung cancer. It has been discovered that patients with advanced non-small cell lung cancer do better when this combination is used. These combinations offer a multimodal approach to cancer treatment by focusing on various pathways implicated in tumor growth.

Biomarkers and Personalized Medical Care:

Personalized medicine—where medications are customized for individual patients based on their unique genetic makeup—is becoming more and more important in the treatment of cancer. In this paradigm, avastin is essential. Scientists are trying to find particular biomarkers that can indicate which patients will respond best to Avastin treatment. In this way, patients can avoid needless side effects and ensure that Avastin is used properly by giving it to individuals who will benefit from it the most.

New Frontiers in Research:

The influence of avastin on oncology extends beyond its present uses. Further investigation is providing fresh perspectives on its workings and possible uses. Among these newly-emerging fields of study are:

Combinations of Immunotherapies: Avastin in combination with immunotherapies, including checkpoint inhibitors, is an interesting new field of study. By strengthening the immune system's capacity to identify and combat cancer cells, this combination may increase response rates in specific types of cancer.

Neoadjuvant and Adjuvant Therapy: Avastin is being investigated for usage in neoadjuvant (prior to surgery) and adjuvant (after surgery) contexts. The purpose of giving Avastin at these phases is to decrease the size of the tumor before surgery and to target any microscopic disease that may still be present thereafter, increasing the likelihood of a long-term remission.

Pediatric Oncology: Although adult cancer treatment has benefited greatly from Avastin's effectiveness, current research is assessing the drug's potential utility in pediatric oncology, which could lead to a wider range of younger patients receiving treatment.

Obstacles and Prospective Paths:

Avastin has persistent problems despite its potential. Avastin and related targeted therapies are expensive, and efforts are being undertaken to improve the affordability and accessibility of these treatments. Furthermore, research and development efforts are still focused on controlling Avastin's adverse effects and determining which patient populations are most suited for treatment.

In summary, Avastin has significantly changed the way that cancer is treated. Its ability to block angiogenesis has established a standard for targeted cancer treatments. Avastin's position in the future of cancer treatment remains crucial as research tackles obstacles and opens up new avenues. It gives patients hope and advances oncology toward more individualized and efficient ways to fight this complicated and deadly illness.

CHAPTER 13

Research and Development: The Avastin Legacy Insights into ongoing research and improvements in Avastin-related treatments.

First of all,

Beyond its groundbreaking introduction, Avastin has left a lasting legacy in the field of oncology through continued research and development. This chapter explores the most recent advancements and insights in the field of Avastin-related treatments, delving into the ever-changing environment of this field.

Sustained Progress in Treatments Associated with Avastin:

Research is aimed at expanding on the success of Avastin, which has opened a new chapter in the treatment of cancer. Avastin's legacy is ever-evolving and can be accessed through the following channels:

1. Increasing Indications

Although avastin was first licensed for the treatment of particular cancer types, research is extending its uses. To increase its influence in the fight against cancer, clinical trials are investigating its effectiveness in a range of malignancies, including glioblastoma and ovarian cancer. The goal of these ongoing trials is to give patients with a variety of cancer types greater options.

2. Discovering Biomarkers:

Cancer treatment is at the forefront thanks to personalized medicine. The goal of research is to find biomarkers that indicate how a patient will react to Avastin. Identification of the most likely beneficiaries allows for the customization of treatment for optimal efficacy and minimal side effects.

Three. Accurate Targeting:

One important aspect of Avastin's legacy is the development of more targeted medicines. Researchers are trying to find novel pharmacological targets and mechanisms in order to improve the accuracy of treatments connected to Avastin. This could result in treatments that block angiogenesis even more potently and precisely.

Complementary Therapies:

Combining Avastin with immunotherapy, chemotherapy, and other targeted therapies is becoming more and more common. The goal of research is to determine the best combinations to enhance patient outcomes. These combinations are intended to disrupt different cancer growth pathways at the same time by acting on many fronts.

Investigating Mechanisms of Resistance:

Understanding why some patients eventually become resistant to Avastin is an important topic of research. Scientists hope to devise ways around or above this obstacle by exploring the systems that underlie resistance. This could entail creating novel medications or therapy plans.

Children's Oncology:

Current studies are also investigating the use of Avastin in pediatric oncology. Since children with cancer frequently require different forms of treatment, research is being done on the usage of Avastin in this patient population to offer more individualized care and better results.

Prospective Routes:

The continual story of progress and hope in the fight against cancer is Avastin's legacy. Future developments in Avastin-related therapies are very promising, with an emphasis on boosting accuracy, extending the drug's useful life, and improving patient outcomes.

In summary:

The legacy of Avastin is not limited to the past; it is still influencing cancer treatment in the present and the future. Its uses are being expanded, its accuracy is being improved, and it will continue to be an essential tool in the oncologist's toolbox thanks to ongoing research and development. The quest for better options for cancer patients is exemplified by the voyage of discovery in Avastin-related medicines, which gives them hope and the possibility of better outcomes.

Section 14

More specific research and advancements in therapies related to Avastin:

1. Avastin with Immune Checkpoint Inhibitors:

Combining Avastin with immune checkpoint inhibitors (ICIs) like nivolumab and pembrolizumab is a major field of research. These treatments function by directing the immune system's attack on cancerous cells. Since Avastin can aid in normalizing the vasculature of the tumor and enhancing immune cell infiltration, the combination therapy aims to enhance the immunological response. Research is being done on the potential synergy between these treatments for a number of cancer types, including some lung malignancies and renal cell carcinoma.

2. Alternative Anti-Angiogenic Treatments to Avastin:

Even though Avastin was the first anti-angiogenic treatment, research is still being done to create other medications that target angiogenesis via various methods. Some of the drawbacks of Avastin, like the emergence of resistance, might be resolved by these innovative treatments. Researchers hope to expand the anti-angiogenic toolkit and maybe enhance patient outcomes by doing so.

Three. Targeted agents combined with combination therapies:

Apart from immune checkpoint inhibitors, the combination of Avastin with other targeted therapy is being investigated. For example, it is used in conjunction with EGFR inhibitors such as cetuximab or panitumumab to treat colorectal cancer. Multiple routes are targeted by these combinations, enhancing the likelihood of success and postponing resistance. One interesting direction in the ongoing development of medicines connected to Avastin is the continuous exploration of optimal combinations.

4. Using Patient Stratification to Find Biomarkers:

Personalized medicine places great emphasis on the discovery of biomarkers that facilitate the identification of patients most likely to benefit from Avastin. New biomarkers, such as genetic mutations or particular protein expressions, are being discovered by scientists through continuing study, and these markers might help inform therapy choices. By using this method, Avastin is given to the people who will benefit from it the most.

5. Mechanisms of Resistance and Overcoming It:

It is crucial to do research to determine the causes of patients' Avastin resistance. Through identifying the underlying mechanisms of resistance, scientists can create solutions to get around or beyond this problem. This could entail creating novel medications that target different pathways or creative treatment plans.

6. Combination Treatments for Childhood Oncology:

Research on Avastin is also being pursued in the field of pediatric oncology. The use of Avastin in pediatric cancer patients is being investigated since childhood cancer frequently presents differently and presents with new obstacles. Clinical trials are evaluating its effectiveness and safety in younger individuals, potentially leading to more individualized treatment plans.

6. Improved Systems for Drug Delivery:

Research on innovative drug delivery systems is an additional topic. Researchers are looking for ways to more effectively deliver Avastin and comparable therapies to the tumor site, which could increase their efficacy and lessen their side effects.

In summary:

Avastin's legacy in oncology is a dynamic tale of advancement and hope. Its uses are being expanded, its precision is being improved, and issues like resistance are being addressed through ongoing research and development. Better outcomes and an enhanced quality of life for patients fighting this difficult disease are anticipated thanks to Avastin's legacy, which is still shaping the landscape of cancer treatment through its exploration of combinations with other treatments, personalization of therapies based on biomarkers, and expansion of its role in pediatric oncology.

CHAPTER 14

Hope Rekindled: Avastin Successes in Clinical Trials Highlighting breakthroughs and positive outcomes in recent trials.

First of all,

In the field of oncology, patients and medical professionals find optimism in the never-ending search for more potent cancer treatments. Leading these efforts has been the innovative anti-angiogenic treatment, avastin (bevacizumab). This chapter highlights Avastin's recent clinical trial accomplishments, highlighting the discoveries and encouraging results that give hope for the fight against cancer.

Novel developments in clinical trials:

Avastin has shown exceptional promise in recent clinical trials, changing the standard of care for a variety of cancer types. Among the noteworthy accomplishments are:

1. Breast Cancer:

Clinical trials have demonstrated that in individuals with advanced ovarian cancer, Avastin greatly increases progression-free survival when coupled with chemotherapy. Because of this accomplishment, Avastin has been approved for the treatment of ovarian cancer, giving women who are battling this difficult disease fresh hope.

2. Multiform Glioblastoma:

In oncology, glioblastoma, a very aggressive brain tumor, has shown to be a tough foe. The clinical trials with Avastin have provided some hope. Studies have shown that glioblastoma patients' quality of life and survival can be increased by adding Avastin to normal therapies.

Three. Cancer of the Renal Cells:

Avastin-based combination treatments have shown to be very beneficial for patients with renal cell carcinoma. Improved progression-free survival and overall survival rates have been seen in clinical trials, demonstrating the potential role of Avastin as a pivotal element in the management of this kidney cancer.

4. Chest Cancer:

Research on avastin's function in advanced non-small cell lung cancer (NSCLC) has also been conducted in large quantities. Clinical trials have shown that Avastin is a useful addition to the treatment arsenal for lung cancer, as it can improve progression-free survival and overall survival when paired with chemotherapy.

5. Hepatocellular Cancer:

Promising results have been obtained from ongoing clinical trials investigating the role of Avastin in colorectal cancer. When combined with chemotherapy, this therapy has increased the survival rate of patients with metastatic colorectal cancer and is now an essential component of the treatment plan.

6. Current Investigations in Pediatric Oncology:

Clinical trials are evaluating the safety and effectiveness of Avastin in children with different forms of cancer in the field of pediatric oncology. These trials give young cancer patients hope for better results and more individualized therapy options.

In summary:

In the field of oncology, Avastin's recent clinical trial achievements are a ray of hope. These discoveries have revised treatment guidelines and broadened the range of cancer types for which Avastin can be used. Avastin's influence on the direction of cancer treatment is still great as research into the disease continues to yield new discoveries and developments. The drug gives patients new hope and a bright future in the never-ending fight against cancer.

Of course, let's take a closer look at Avastin's recent clinical trial triumphs, emphasizing the discoveries and successful outcomes in a range of cancer types:

1. Breast Cancer:

For women fighting ovarian cancer, Avastin's notable progress in clinical trials has changed the game. Studies have demonstrated a significant improvement in progression-free survival when Avastin is taken in addition to conventional treatment. For patients with ovarian cancer, this result is encouraging since it may lead to more strong and long-lasting therapy responses. Additionally, it resulted in Avastin's clearance for the treatment of ovarian cancer in numerous regions, offering a crucial alternative in the battle against this difficult malignancy.

2. Multiform Glioblastoma:

Glioblastoma, one of the deadliest brain cancers, has shown promising outcomes in clinical trials. When included into conventional treatment plans, avastin has demonstrated the ability to increase survival rates and—perhaps more importantly—improve patient quality of life. Glioblastoma patients and their families have hope again because of these trials, which provide a ray of hope against a strong foe.

Three. Cancer of the Renal Cells:

The use of Avastin in clinical trials has revolutionized the field of kidney cancer research. Avastin-based combination treatments have regularly shown improved rates of both overall and progression-free survival. These trials have improved and expanded the therapy choices available to patients with renal cell carcinoma. With its revolutionary role in the fight against kidney cancer, Avastin has given patients afflicted with the disease unprecedented hope.

4. Chest Cancer:

Avastin clinical trials have primarily focused on non-small cell lung cancer (NSCLC). The encouraging findings show that Avastin can considerably raise overall survival and progression-free survival rates when combined with chemotherapy. This advancement offers hope to patients and their families dealing with this difficult diagnosis and is evidence of the effectiveness of Avastin in the treatment of lung cancer.

5. Hepatocellular Cancer:

The efficacy of Avastin in clinical studies for colorectal cancer has been crucial. It has increased the survival rate of individuals with metastatic colorectal cancer when paired with chemotherapy. This accomplishment has changed the landscape of colorectal cancer treatment, giving patients hope and raising the likelihood of a better prognosis.

6. Current Investigations in Pediatric Oncology:

In the field of pediatric oncology, Avastin's safety and effectiveness being investigated in clinical trials provides a ray of hope for kids with different kinds of cancer. These studies show a dedication to offering customized treatment plans and better results to young patients. Avastin's prospective influence on pediatric oncology is evidence of its continuing influence on how cancer care will be provided in the future.

In summary:

For cancer patients with all kinds of cancer, Avastin's recent clinical trial victories are signs of optimism. These discoveries have revolutionized the standards of care, resulting in higher rates of survival, better quality of life, and a resurgence of hope. Avastin's influence on the direction of cancer treatment is still great as new discoveries and developments in the field emerge, giving patients new hope and optimism in the never-ending fight against cancer.

CHAPTER 15

The Human Faces Behind Avastin Research Stories of scientists, clinicians, and patients who have contributed to Avastin's success.

Narratives of patients, doctors, and scientists who have helped make Avastin a success.

Scientists in the Lead

Every medical advancement is the result of experts who devote their entire careers to research and development. The success of Avastin is not unusual. The following are a few of the trailblazing scientists that have contributed to the creation of this innovative treatment:

Napoleone Ferrara: A well-known researcher on cancer, Dr. Ferrara was instrumental in the identification of VEGF, a protein that is essential for the development of blood vessels in tumors. His ground-breaking research served as a catalyst for the creation of Avastin. His unwavering commitment to deciphering the complexities of cancer biology has had a profound effect on cancer treatment.

Joan Folkman: Known as the "mother of angiogenesis," Dr. Folkman's research on the function of angiogenesis in the development of cancer and her partnership with Dr. Ferrara were crucial in the creation of Avastin. Her innovative theories revolutionized the study of cancer and advanced targeted treatments like Avastin.

Susan Desmond-Hellmann: As the leader of Genentech during the creation of Avastin, Dr. Desmond-Hellmann was instrumental in the process. Avastin was brought from the lab to the clinic thanks to her leadership and dedication to providing patients with cutting-edge cancer treatments. Her foresight had a major influence on Avastin's development and effects on cancer treatment.

Honorable Physicians

Front-line clinicians have played a crucial role in the success of Avastin. In addition to providing the treatment, they have carried out clinical trials, obtaining important information and understanding. A few tales stick out:

Dr. George Sledge: Sledge is an oncologist and researcher who participated in clinical trials for breast cancer using Avastin. Though it was not widely approved, his work was crucial in examining Avastin's potential for treating breast cancer. His commitment to developing more effective therapies for breast cancer patients has a long-lasting effect.

Dr. Mark Gilbert is a neuro-oncologist who has been actively involved in clinical trials for brain cancers using Avastin. His dedication to investigating novel treatments for people with glioblastoma multiforme and glioma has given hope to those battling these severe malignancies.

Dr. Herbert Hurwitz: Leading clinical trials to look at the usage of Avastin in colorectal cancer, Dr. Hurwitz is a medical oncologist. His work significantly prolonged the lives of many patients by making Avastin the accepted standard of care for this kind of cancer.

Fearless Patients

The experiences of clinical trial participants, whose resiliency and optimism motivated scientists and medical professionals, are essential to the Avastin journey. These people cleared the path for future patients to get cutting-edge therapies in addition to making significant contributions to the development of Avastin. Among their tales are the following:

Anna: After receiving a colon cancer diagnosis, Anna signed up for an Avastin clinical trial. Her reaction to the medication, prolonged survival, and enhanced quality of life served as evidence of Avastin's practical benefits.

David: Despite having glioblastoma, David took part in an Avastin clinical trial. Despite receiving a tragic diagnosis, his amazing response to the medication demonstrated the promise of Avastin in the treatment of brain tumors and sparked optimism.

Maria: Maria's experience with ovarian cancer brought her to the attention of researchers studying Avastin in a clinical trial. Her experience served as evidence of Avastin's advantages in the treatment of this difficult cancer kind.

These are only a handful of the innumerable patients whose bravery and readiness to take part in clinical trials made Avastin a success possible. Their experiences serve as a monument to the ability of innovation and research to change the face of cancer care.

Avastin has progressed from a notion in the laboratory to a life-changing medication in the clinic thanks to the real faces behind the research, including the brilliant scientists, the committed physicians, and the brave patients. Generations of researchers, physicians, and patients have been motivated by their steadfast dedication and common optimism, which has paved the way to improved cancer care. The remarkable potential that can be achieved when science, commitment, and human spirit come together in the fight against cancer is demonstrated by the legacy of Avastin.

Narratives of patients, doctors, and scientists who have helped make Avastin a success.

Scientists in the Lead

Every medical advancement is the result of experts who devote their entire careers to research and development. The success of Avastin is not unusual. The following are a few of the trailblazing scientists that have contributed to the creation of this innovative treatment:

Napoleone Ferrara: A well-known researcher on cancer, Dr. Ferrara was instrumental in the identification of VEGF, a protein that is essential for the development of blood vessels in tumors. His ground-breaking research served as a catalyst for the creation of Avastin. Dr. Ferrara is regarded as a leader in the field of cancer treatment because of his unwavering commitment to deciphering the complexities of cancer biology and angiogenesis.

Joan Folkman: Known as the "mother of angiogenesis," Dr. Folkman's research on the function of angiogenesis in the development of cancer and her partnership with Dr. Ferrara were crucial in the creation of Avastin. Her innovative theories revolutionized the study of cancer and advanced targeted treatments like Avastin. Dr. Folkman's seminal contributions to cancer therapy science have made a lasting impression.

Susan Desmond-Hellmann: As the leader of Genentech during the creation of Avastin, Dr. Desmond-Hellmann was instrumental in the process. Avastin was brought from the lab to the clinic thanks to her leadership and dedication to providing patients with cutting-edge cancer treatments. The development of Avastin and its effects on cancer treatment were greatly influenced by Dr. Desmond-Hellmann's vision, and her legacy in oncology is still felt today.

Honorable Physicians

Front-line clinicians have played a crucial role in the success of Avastin. In addition to providing the treatment, they have carried out clinical trials, obtaining important information and understanding. A few tales stick out:

Dr. George Sledge: Sledge is an oncologist and researcher who participated in clinical trials for breast cancer using Avastin. Though it was not widely approved, his work was crucial in examining Avastin's potential for treating breast cancer. A long-lasting influence on the profession, Dr. Sledge's commitment to improving treatments for breast cancer patients continues to motivate researchers.

Dr. Mark Gilbert is a neuro-oncologist who has been actively involved in clinical trials for brain cancers using Avastin. His dedication to investigating novel treatments for people with glioblastoma multiforme and glioma has given hope to those battling these severe malignancies. Because to Dr. Gilbert's unwavering commitment to helping patients with brain tumors, our understanding of these difficult conditions has changed.

Dr. Herbert Hurwitz: Leading clinical trials to look at the usage of Avastin in colorectal cancer, Dr. Hurwitz is a medical oncologist. His work significantly prolonged the lives of many patients by making Avastin the accepted standard of care for this kind of cancer. A lasting legacy in clinical research and colorectal cancer treatment has been established by Dr. Hurwitz's efforts.

Fearless Patients

The experiences of clinical trial participants, whose resiliency and optimism motivated scientists and medical professionals, are essential to the Avastin journey. These people cleared the path for future patients to get cutting-edge therapies in addition to making significant contributions to the development of Avastin. Among their tales are the following:

Anna: After receiving a colon cancer diagnosis, Anna signed up for an Avastin clinical trial. Her reaction to the medication, prolonged survival, and enhanced quality of life served as evidence of Avastin's practical benefits. Anna's experience serves as an example of how cutting-edge medicines can significantly improve patients' lives.

David: Despite having glioblastoma, David took part in an Avastin clinical trial. Despite receiving a tragic diagnosis, his amazing response to the medication demonstrated the promise of Avastin in the treatment of brain tumors and sparked optimism. David's narrative serves as a tribute to the bravery of individuals who actively engage in clinical trials to further the treatment of cancer.

Maria: Maria's experience with ovarian cancer brought her to the attention of researchers studying Avastin in a clinical trial. Her experience served as evidence of Avastin's advantages in the treatment of this difficult cancer kind. Maria's narrative demonstrates how patients influence the field of cancer treatment and give hope to those going through comparable difficulties.

These are only a handful of the innumerable patients whose bravery and readiness to take part in clinical trials made Avastin a success possible. Their experiences serve as a monument to the ability of innovation and research to change the face of cancer care. They serve as a reminder of how closely the lives and experiences of actual people affect the advancements made in the field of oncology.

Avastin has progressed from a notion in the laboratory to a life-changing medication in the clinic thanks to the real faces behind the research, including the brilliant scientists, the committed physicians, and the brave patients. Generations of researchers, physicians, and patients have been motivated by their steadfast dedication and common optimism, which has paved the way to improved cancer care. The remarkable potential that can be achieved when science, commitment, and human spirit come together in the fight against cancer is demonstrated by the legacy of Avastin. All those who are committed to the fight against cancer get encouragement from their stories.

CHAPTER 16

The Global Impact of Avastin
Examining Avastin's role in the
international fight against cancer.

analyzing Avastin's contribution to the global cancer epidemic.

Worldwide Reach

Avastin is a major participant in the global fight against cancer because of its far-reaching effects on cancer care. Its transformation from an innovative discovery to a well-known treatment has had a significant impact on the global healthcare scene.

Nations, Developed and Developing

Patients in developed and developing countries have benefited from Avastin's ability to remove obstacles in the way of receiving state-of-the-art cancer treatment. It has become a crucial component of cancer care in affluent nations, increasing survival rates and improving many patients' quality of life.

The availability of Avastin has significantly closed treatment gaps for cancer in underdeveloped nations. Patients who had few options before now have access to it because to partnerships and initiatives. It has an incalculable positive effect on patients in these areas, providing a glimmer of hope amidst hardship.

Worldwide Clinical Studies

The use of avastin in therapeutic practice is not the only aspect of its global influence. It has played a major role in international clinical trials, enabling patients from all backgrounds to take part in state-of-the-art studies. Our knowledge of Avastin's effectiveness in treating different cancer kinds and populations has improved as a result of these trials.

Resource Difficulties

In many regions of the world, the fight against cancer faces significant obstacles due to a lack of resources and healthcare inequities. The story of Avastin highlights the significance of resolving these inequalities and coming up with creative ways to guarantee that even the most marginalized groups have access to cutting-edge cancer treatments.

Cooperation and Information Sharing

The collaborative efforts and knowledge exchange between healthcare professionals, researchers, and politicians from other nations is another indication of Avastin's global influence. Exploiting Avastin's potential to its fullest potential is what motivates the global community to work together to end cancer.

Upcoming Prospects

Avastin's importance in the global fight against cancer is expected to grow as the struggle progresses. Future research, multinational partnerships, and creative thinking will determine how much of an impact Avastin has on a worldwide scale.

The worldwide influence of Avastin bears witness to the revolutionary capacity of medical discoveries and the collective resolve of the global community to improve cancer treatment. It is a wonderful example of the strength of science, teamwork, and unshakable commitment in the global fight against cancer. The legacy of Avastin is still being created, which serves as a reminder that the fight against cancer is an international effort in which we can all work together to improve the lives of innumerable patients worldwide.

Worldwide Reach

Avastin is a major participant in the global fight against cancer because of its far-reaching effects on cancer care. Its transformation from an innovative discovery to a well-known treatment has had a significant impact on the global healthcare scene.

Nations, Developed and Developing

Patients in developed and developing countries have benefited from Avastin's ability to remove obstacles in the way of receiving state-of-the-art cancer treatment. It has become a crucial component of cancer care in affluent nations, increasing survival rates and improving many patients' quality of life.

Avastin has completely changed the way that many cancer types are treated in affluent nations with well-established healthcare systems. Patients' lives have been considerably extended by its usage in conjunction with chemotherapy and other targeted medicines, giving many with depressing diagnoses fresh hope.

Avastin has been essential in filling important gaps in cancer treatment in developing countries where healthcare resources can be scarce. Patients who had few options before now have access to it thanks to collaborations and initiatives by governments, pharmaceutical firms, and other groups. It has an incalculable positive effect on patients in these areas, providing a glimmer of hope amidst hardship. Avastin has shown promise in bringing cutting-edge cancer treatments to underprivileged communities by reducing worldwide disparities in cancer care.

Worldwide Clinical Studies

The use of avastin in therapeutic practice is not the only aspect of its global influence. It has played a major role in international clinical trials, enabling patients from various locations and backgrounds to take part in state-of-the-art studies. The aforementioned trials have contributed to our comprehension of Avastin's effectiveness in many disease kinds and people, underscoring the need of adopting a global viewpoint in cancer research.

In addition to advancing the science, international clinical trials have made it possible for patients anywhere in the globe to get cutting-edge medicines, no matter where they live. This international approach to research guarantees that patients from different locations and cultural backgrounds can take advantage of the most recent discoveries.

Resource Difficulties

In many regions of the world, the fight against cancer faces significant obstacles due to a lack of resources and healthcare inequities. The story of Avastin highlights the significance of resolving these inequalities and coming up with creative ways to guarantee that even the most marginalized groups have access to cutting-edge cancer treatments. This entails getting beyond barriers pertaining to healthcare access, infrastructure, and treatment costs.

The widespread effects of Avastin underscore the necessity of more extensive global health initiatives to address resource gaps that may restrict the accessibility of ground-breaking treatments. One of the key objectives of the international campaign against cancer is still to be able to provide cutting-edge therapies to every country in the globe.

Cooperation and Information Sharing

The collaborative efforts and knowledge exchange between healthcare professionals, researchers, and politicians from other nations is another indication of Avastin's global influence. Exploiting Avastin's potential to its fullest potential is what motivates the global community to work together to end cancer. International cooperation has sped up research and the exchange of best practices, creating a worldwide network of professionals committed to enhancing cancer treatment.

Upcoming Prospects

Avastin's importance in the global fight against cancer is expected to grow as the struggle progresses. Future research, multinational partnerships, and creative thinking will determine how much of an impact Avastin has on a worldwide scale. We may expect even more notable developments in Avastin usage in the years to come, in terms of both its accessibility and its range of uses.

The worldwide influence of Avastin bears witness to the revolutionary capacity of medical discoveries and the collective resolve of the global community to improve cancer treatment.

It is a wonderful example of the strength of science, teamwork, and unshakable commitment in the global fight against cancer. The legacy of Avastin is still being created, which serves as a reminder that the fight against cancer is an international effort in which we can all work together to improve the lives of innumerable patients worldwide. Avastin's worldwide influence is a reflection of our shared dedication to ending cancer and providing hope to people everywhere.

Chapter 17

Navigating Insurance and Financial Challenges Providing advice on dealing with the financial aspects of Avastin treatment.

First of all,

Managing a severe medical condition such as Avastin treatment can provide both physical and mental difficulties. Nevertheless, the financial strain this journey may place on patients and their families is one of the frequently disregarded parts of it. We will offer helpful guidance in this chapter on navigating the tricky insurance landscape and monetary obstacles while receiving Avastin treatment.

Comprehending The Costs of Avastin Treatment:

It's critical to comprehend the expenses related to Avastin treatment before delving into the intricacies of insurance. Since Avastin is a biologic medication, it is important to understand the entire cost structure, including the medication itself, its administration, and any associated medical services.

Insurance Protection:

Examine Your coverage: To begin, go over your health insurance coverage in detail. Recognize what costs linked with Avastin are covered, such as the medication, visits to the doctor, hospital stays, and any related services.

Talk to Your Insurer: Make contact with your insurance company to go over your course of treatment. Make detailed inquiries on the scope of coverage, any prerequisites for pre-authorization, and the procedure for submitting claims.

Appeal Denials: Keep trying if your insurance company refuses to pay for Avastin or associated costs. A lengthy but potentially successful appeals process is offered by several insurance companies. Your physician can frequently assist by supplying the required records and explanations.

Programs for Financial Assistance:
The company that makes Avastin, Genentech, provides patients who qualify with financial aid programs that might lower the cost of the

medication. Examine your eligibility for these programs, then collaborate with your medical team to submit an application.

Organizations that Promote Patients:
Numerous patient advocacy organizations offer assistance and services to people undergoing costly medical treatments. They can provide you with options for financial support and emotional support when you travel.

Planning finances and creating a budget:
Effective cost management can be achieved by developing a financial strategy and budget tailored to your course of treatment. Think about things like co-pays, deductibles, and travel costs if your treatment facility is out of town.

Programs for Prescription Assistance:

Look into foundations or prescription assistance programs that might be able to assist with the cost of Avastin or other prescription drugs. Certain regimens are tailored to individual diseases and can offer substantial alleviation.

Protections and Legal Rights:
Understand your legal rights regarding insurance coverage. Certain state and federal statutes offer cancer patients rights that guarantee them access to essential treatments.

In summary:
It might be difficult to manage the financial implications of Avastin treatment, but it's important to avoid adding financial worries to an already trying period. You can lessen some of the financial strain related to Avastin therapy by being aware of your insurance coverage, getting

financial aid, and making a sound financial plan. Recall that you are not alone on this road and that there are groups and resources available to help you at every turn.

Comprehending The Costs of Avastin Treatment:

Understanding the breakdown of the costs associated with Avastin treatment is essential before you can manage the financial obstacles that come with it. Being a biologic medication, avastin is often expensive. Here's a closer look at the things you ought to think about:

Cost Components: There are multiple components to the costs related to receiving treatment with Avastin. These include the price of the medication itself, which varies according on how often and at what dose it is taken. In addition, there are costs associated with receiving medical services, like hospital stays, doctor visits, and lab testing.

Treatment Length: Avastin therapy is frequently given in cycles, lasting a few months. You can more precisely estimate the total costs of your therapy if you know how long it is expected to take.

Insurance Protection:

A crucial component of handling the financial side of your therapy is understanding insurance. Here's a closer look at handling insurance:

Review Your Policy: Go over your health insurance policy paperwork carefully, making sure to read the parts on outpatient services, biologic medications, and cancer therapies in particular. Take note of any restrictions, limitations, or prerequisites.

Talk with Your Insurer: It's a good idea to speak with your insurance company as soon as possible. Tell them about your treatment plan and make specific inquiries about insurance. For example, find out if pre-authorization is necessary, if Avastin itself is covered, and what steps you need to do to guarantee that your claims are handled efficiently.

Appeal Denials: Occasionally, insurance companies may initially refuse to pay for specific costs associated with using Avastin. If this occurs, persevere. To contest denials, one can use the appeals process offered by many insurers. Your oncologist and other members of your healthcare team can frequently supply the paperwork and medical explanations required to back up your appeal.

Programs for Financial Assistance:

When it comes to paying for Avastin treatment, financial assistance programs might offer significant comfort. Further information on these programs can be found here:

Manufacturer Programs: Avastin's maker, Genentech, provides qualified people with patient support programs. The out-of-pocket expenses for the medication can be greatly decreased with these schemes. Examine your eligibility and, in collaboration with your medical team, submit an application.

Organizations that Promote Patients:

Patient advocacy groups are essential in assisting people in overcoming the financial obstacles associated with cancer treatments. They provide a variety of tools and assistance:

Resource Assistance: These groups frequently have databases on foundations, financial aid schemes, and other resources that can lessen the cost of Avastin treatment.

Emotional Support: Managing a major illness and the monetary difficulties that come with it can be emotionally taxing. Patient advocacy organizations can help you get through this tough period by putting you in touch with counseling and support groups.

Planning finances and creating a budget:

Developing a financial strategy and budget tailored to your Avastin treatment can significantly improve your financial management:

Incorporate All fees: If the treatment facility is far away, your budget should account for probable housing as well as indirect fees like travel to and from the facility. These should be included in addition to the direct medical expenses.

Emergency Fund: To pay for unforeseen expenses that might occur during your treatment path, think about creating or accessing an emergency fund.

Programs for Prescription Assistance:

Examine the foundations and prescription assistance programs that are available:

Programs for Particular Illnesses: Certain organizations concentrate on particular illnesses, such as cancer. They might offer financial support for Avastin or similar drugs.

Application Process: Be ready to submit documentation of your financial status, including income, costs, and medical bills, when submitting an application for such programs.

Protections and Legal Rights:

Dealing with insurance and financial difficulties may require you to be aware of your legal rights:

Patient Bill of Rights: Become acquainted with the Patient Bill of Rights, which delineates the safeguards and privileges available to patients receiving medical care, including cancer treatment.

State Laws: Be advised that certain states may offer cancer sufferers extra guarantees and protections. These regulations frequently mandate that insurers pay for particular surgeries or treatments.

In conclusion, managing the cost of Avastin therapy necessitates a thorough strategy. You may better handle the financial parts of your journey by being aware of your legal rights, making a budget, understanding your insurance coverage, and asking for financial assistance.

Remind yourself that you are not alone in this difficult time and that there are many organizations and resources available to assist you.

CHAPTER 18

Advocacy and Support: Patient Communities and Organizations Recognizing the role of advocacy groups in supporting Avastin patients.

First of all,

It can be difficult and lonely to manage a medical condition like Avastin medication. Advocacy groups and patient networks frequently provide consolation and crucial assistance to patients and their families. We will discuss the vital function these groups play in helping Avastin patients as well as how they can help to ease the trip in this chapter.

The Function of Lobbying Groups:

Advocacy groups are essential in providing multiple forms of support to people receiving Avastin treatment.

Knowledge and Education: These groups offer current resources and information regarding Avastin, its adverse effects, and available treatments. Patients can obtain useful educational resources to help them comprehend their illness and make wise decisions.

Emotional Support: Managing a life-threatening illness can be extremely taxing on the emotions. Advocacy groups provide a forum for patients to establish connections with like-minded individuals. This sense of belonging can lessen feelings of loneliness and offer consolation and support when things are hard.

Advocacy and Awareness: A large number of patient advocacy organizations engage in active advocacy on behalf of patients' rights, treatment access, and greater public knowledge of the illnesses they represent. They seek to advance research and sculpt policy in ways that benefit the patient population.

Financial Assistance: To assist patients with the cost of therapies like Avastin, certain advocacy groups offer financial support programs. The financial load can be considerably reduced by these initiatives.

Patient Communities' Assistance:

Peer support: Online and offline patient communities bring together people on similar treatment paths. A sense of community and solace can be gained from discussing experiences and coping mechanisms with peers.

Expert Access: A lot of patient groups want medical professionals to respond to inquiries and concerns. Patients may receive reliable information and answers to their questions about medicine thanks to this direct connection to medical specialists.

Choosing a Course of therapy: Patients frequently encounter difficulties choosing a course of therapy and navigating the healthcare system. Patient forums can help by offering advice and exchanging best practices for dealing with these issues.

Lobbying for Change: Certain patient communities actively support policy changes and research funding in addition to offering assistance. Their combined voice has the power to change healthcare laws and raise standards of treatment.

Understanding the Significance of Support and Advocacy:

Patients taking Avastin should understand the importance of patient communities and advocacy groups in their journey:

Maintaining Knowledge: Having a thorough understanding of your illness and available treatments is empowering. You can obtain useful information from patient communities and advocacy groups to assist you in making decisions.

Creating a Support Network: You can get a lot of emotional support from people who are in similar situations as you. These communities' common experiences can foster enduring friendships and a feeling of community.

Advocating for Change: These groups can provide you with the information and resources you need to advocate for change if you believe that there are gaps in the healthcare system or that getting treatment is difficult.

Obtaining Financial Assistance: Investigate the financial aid schemes that advocacy organizations offer without holding back. The journey can be made considerably less stressful by lowering the cost of treatment.

To sum up, patient communities and advocacy organizations are essential to the lives of people using Avastin. They give access to financial aid, advocacy, information, and emotional support. Patients taking Avastin can enhance their general well-being and more effectively manage their medication by appreciating the importance of these organizations and actively interacting with them.

Of course, let's examine the significance of patient networks and advocacy groups for Avastin users in more detail:

The Function of Lobbying Groups:

Knowledge and Instruction:
Patients taking Avastin can benefit greatly from the information and educational resources

provided by advocacy groups. They inform patients on new research, possible side effects, and the most recent developments in the Avastin treatment. Patients are better equipped to make knowledgeable decisions about their treatment options and to have informed conversations with their healthcare providers thanks to this information.

Emotional Assistance:

The emotional support advocacy groups offer is among their greatest advantages. Managing a severe medical illness such as Avastin therapy can be emotionally and psychologically taxing. These support groups provide a secure environment where patients can talk to people who understand their struggles and express their worries, anxieties, and victories. This sense of belonging lowers feelings of loneliness and may enhance mental health.

Awareness and Advocacy:

Numerous advocacy groups actively work to promote patient rights and greater public understanding of the illnesses they represent. To guarantee that patients have access to the finest care possible, they collaborate with legislators, medical professionals, and members of the public. Their work may result in better insurance coverage, easier access to cutting-edge therapies, and a deeper comprehension of the difficulties that patients encounter.

Financial Support:

Some advocacy organizations provide financial assistance programs in recognition of the financial burden that Avastin treatment can have on patients and their families. Patients can receive assistance from these programs with Avastin-related expenditures, such as co-pays and deductibles. These initiatives help to enhance treatment adherence and general well-being by easing some of the financial strain.

Patient Communities' Assistance:

Peer Assistance:

Online or in person, patient networks bring together people undergoing similar medical treatments. Engaging with others who have undergone similar experiences can foster a feeling of unity and mutual comprehension. By exchanging helpful tips and emotional support, patients can make the journey easier to handle.

Obtaining Expertise:

Patient communities frequently organize conferences or webinars including medical experts with expertise in Avastin therapy. Patients can ask questions and voice concerns about their illness, treatment, and side effects since they have direct access to professionals. It guarantees that patients obtain accurate and trustworthy information to help them make decisions.

Getting Around Treatment:
It can be quite difficult to navigate the healthcare system, comprehend technical medical terms, and handle treatment logistics. Patient communities frequently offer advice on these matters. These communities provide helpful assistance in the form of suggestions for the greatest treatment facilities, strategies for

handling side effects, and guidance on leading a healthy lifestyle while undergoing treatment.

Organizing for Reform:

In addition to receiving one-on-one assistance, some patient communities actively advocate for funding for research and legislative changes. Their combined voice has the power to change healthcare laws, increase public awareness of Avastin patients' needs, and enhance the standard of care and available treatments.

Understanding the Significance of Support and Advocacy:

Remaining Up to Date:

Patients on Avastin should benefit from the abundance of information offered by advocacy organizations. Patients can take an active role in their healthcare decisions and act as an advocate for themselves by being knowledgeable about their disease, available treatments, and any possible negative effects.

Creating a Network of Support:
The emotional journey associated with taking Avastin might be lonely. Getting involved in advocacy groups and patient communities can help patients build a network of support where they can talk about their struggles, victories, and anxieties. These relationships frequently last past the course of treatment, resulting in enduring friendships and a deep sense of community.

Pushing for Reform:
Patients on Avastin can be change agents as well as passive beneficiaries of care. Patients can positively impact healthcare legislation and the

patient experience by actively engaging in advocacy initiatives, such as bringing attention to the ailment and its treatment issues.

Getting Financial Support:
Investigate the financial aid schemes offered by advocacy organizations without holding back. These initiatives aim to lower the cost of care and increase its accessibility. Patients can free themselves from the burden of money worries and concentrate on their health by using these tools.

To sum up, patient networks and advocacy groups provide a wealth of resources for Avastin users, ranging from financial aid and advocacy to knowledge and emotional support. Patients can improve their quality of life and face their treatment path with more resilience and confidence by actively participating with these groups.

Chapter 19

Lessons from the Avastin Journey
Reflecting on the broader lessons
learned from the Avastin story.

First of all,

The Avastin journey includes not only the actual medical treatment but also the important life lessons that patients and their families can take away from their experiences. We will discuss the larger takeaways from the Avastin narrative in this chapter. These takeaways go beyond the confines of a particular treatment and could influence our perceptions of resilience, healthcare, and the human spirit.

1. The Influence of Medical Developments:

The Avastin narrative highlights the remarkable potential of medical progress. As a biologic medication, avastin has revolutionized the way that many tumors are treated. The significance of continuous research and innovation in the healthcare sector is the lesson to be learned from this. It's evidence of what can be accomplished when medicine and science collaborate to enhance patient outcomes.

2. The Value of Prompt Detection

Avastin is frequently utilized in the latter phases of cancer treatment; nonetheless, its effectiveness serves as a reminder of the significance of prompt detection and action. Cancer therapies can be greatly impacted by routine screenings and knowledge of possible symptoms. The Avastin trip emphasizes how important it is to identify medical disorders early on, when they are more manageable.

Three. The Human Spirit's Adaptability:
Patients on Avastin and their families have exhibited remarkable fortitude amidst a difficult medical path. The teachings presented are not limited to medicine; they also touch on the human spirit's amazing capacity to endure, adjust, and find hope in the face of extreme adversity.

4. The Function of Support Systems:
The Avastin experience serves as a timely reminder of the need of support systems, which include friends, family, advocacy organizations, and medical professionals. It serves as an example of how group assistance may make a path easier to travel. The takeaway from this

experience is to develop and depend on a support network when dealing with health issues.

5. Engagement of Patients and Advocacy:

Patients on Avastin frequently develop into advocates for both their own and other people's healthcare. This trip has shown us that patients are not silent and can actively engage in advocacy, research, and healthcare decision-making. Policies that enhance the patient experience can be influenced and changed by patients.

6. Handling the Healthcare Complexities:

The Avastin tale demonstrates the intricacies of healthcare systems, encompassing everything from insurance and coverage concerns to treatment scheduling. In this confusing environment, patients and their families frequently develop into skilled navigators. This illustrates how crucial it is to be knowledgeable about healthcare and the nuances of the system in order to make wise decisions.

6. Savoring the Moments in Life:
Having a major medical illness can alter one's outlook on life. Patients on Avastin frequently learn to respect life, cherishing time spent with loved ones and concentrating on what really matters. The voyage reminds us that happiness and purpose may be found in life, despite hardship.

8. The Possibility of Optimism and Fortitude:
The story of Avastin shows that perseverance and optimism are possible even in the face of severe medical difficulties. Families, healthcare

professionals, and patients all exhibit unflinching resolve and hope for better times to come. The lesson is that the healing process can benefit greatly from the presence of hope.

9. The Constant Search for a Cure:
Even if it works well, the vastin therapy cannot treat cancer. This emphasizes the continuous necessity for investigation and efforts to discover long-term treatment for illnesses. The trip inspires us to keep funding medical innovation and research.

In summary, the Avastin journey is a monument to the resiliency of the human spirit, the value of early discovery, and the strength of activism and support, in addition to being a tale of medical therapy. It serves as a reminder to value life, participate in healthcare decisions, and keep searching for medical breakthroughs that will enhance the quality of life for patients and their families. We are all inspired and wisedened by the more general teachings discovered on our trip.

Of course, let's explore more deeply the more general lessons that the Avastin expedition can teach us:

1. The Influence of Medical Developments:
The Avastin narrative demonstrates the ability of medical progress to significantly improve the prognosis and treatment of cancer and other complicated illnesses. It emphasizes how crucial it is that the healthcare sector continue to invest in, innovate, and do research. This lesson shows us that medicine and science have the power to

significantly enhance and save a great deal of lives.

2. The Value of Prompt Detection

Despite the fact that Avastin is frequently used in advanced stages of cancer, its effectiveness highlights how important early detection is. The Avastin story emphasizes the value of routine screenings and prompt treatment, demonstrating how early detection of medical diseases can significantly improve treatment outcomes and, in certain situations, save lives.

Three. The Human Spirit's Adaptability:

Patients on Avastin and their families are living examples of how remarkably resilient people can be. Their resilience and the power of the human spirit are demonstrated by their capacity to confront the difficulties of a difficult medical journey with bravery, adaptation, and hope. It serves as a reminder that the human spirit can persevere and flourish under the most challenging conditions.

4. The Function of Support Systems:

The Avastin expedition emphasizes how important support systems are. Patients can get emotional, practical, and informational support from these networks, which include medical professionals, advocacy organizations, families, and friends. This lesson emphasizes how crucial it is to build a strong support network and rely on it when navigating health issues.

5. Engagement of Patients and Advocacy:

Patients on Avastin frequently develop a strong advocacy for both their own and other people's healthcare. Their experience shows us that patients are active participants in healthcare decisions, research, and advocacy initiatives rather than passive beneficiaries of care. This lesson promotes patient involvement and the understanding that patients have the ability to significantly influence changes in the healthcare system.

6. Handling the Healthcare Complexities:

The Avastin trip sheds light on the complexities and difficulties found in healthcare systems, such as the difficulties associated with insurance and the logistics of treatment. In navigating these difficulties, patients and their families frequently develop into specialists. This lesson emphasizes how crucial it is to comprehend the healthcare system and be healthcare literate in order to make wise decisions and effectively advocate for others.

6. Savoring the Moments in Life:

Living with a severe illness, like being treated with Avastin, can cause one to reevaluate their outlook on life. Patients frequently learn to value life, cherish time spent with loved ones, and concentrate on what really matters. This lesson encourages us to value the connections and experiences that bring us contentment and to find happiness and purpose in life even in the midst of hardship.

8. The Possibility of Optimism and Fortitude:

The story of Avastin shows that tenacity and hope can exist even in the most trying situations. Patients, along with their family and healthcare personnel, exhibit resoluteness and hope for better times to come. This lesson emphasizes how resilient thinking and hope may be transformative in the healing process.

9. The Constant Search for a Cure:

Avastin is a major improvement in the treatment of cancer, but it is not a cure. This highlights how important it is to keep up research and efforts to identify long-term treatments for illnesses. The Avastin story serves as a timely reminder of the need of funding medical research, creativity, and teamwork in order to enhance patient outcomes and eventually find treatments.

To sum up, the Avastin experience teaches valuable insights that go well beyond the field of medicine. It teaches us about the value of support networks, human resilience, the power of research, the necessity of early identification, the possibility for advocacy, and patient involvement. It also serves as a reminder to treasure the moments in life, hold onto hope and fortitude, and actively participate in the continuous search for medical breakthroughs and treatments. These teachings inspire and educate us all, motivating us to lead meaningful lives and have a beneficial influence on society and healthcare.

CHAPTER 20

The Ongoing Hope: A Brighter Future for Cancer Patients

Concluding the book with a message of hope and a look ahead to the evolving landscape of cancer treatment.

bringing the book to a close with a hopeful message and an outlook on how cancer treatment will develop going forward.

Introduction: As we come to the end of this book, we would like to leave you with a message of optimism and hope for the future of cancer treatment, with an emphasis on the ways that support networks, therapies, and the resilient nature of cancer patients are all changing.

Avastin's path and the larger context of cancer treatment serve as a reminder that, despite ongoing obstacles, hope and advancement are brilliantly visible in the distance.

Developments in Cancer Treatment: Researchers and medical professionals are always coming up with new and creative ways to treat cancer, and this sector is always changing. Precision medicine, immunotherapies, and targeted medicines are revolutionizing the way we treat cancer. These developments give patients new hope for therapies that are more efficient, less intrusive, and more tolerable.

tailored Medicine: The emergence of tailored medicine is one of the most exciting trends. Cancer treatment is becoming more and more patient-specific thanks to developments in genomics and molecular profiling. This makes it possible for more potent and less prone to have adverse treatment outcomes. Treatments tailored to the specific genetic composition of each patient's cancer may be available in the future.

Immunotherapy Breakthroughs: In recent years, immunotherapy, which targets cancer cells by stimulating the body's immune system, has demonstrated impressive efficacy. Numerous malignancies are seeing an increase in treatment options and survival rates because to recent advancements in immunotherapy. Immunotherapies that are even more efficient and widely available may become possible as research progresses.

Patient-Centric Care: A more patient-centric approach to cancer therapy is becoming the norm in the field. When creating treatment programs, patients' interests, values, and quality of life are taken into account more and more. The focus is on giving cancer patients a better overall experience in addition to effective therapies.

The Function of Advocacy and Support:
Cancer patients' lives are still greatly impacted by advocacy groups and support networks, such as those covered in earlier chapters. These organizations provide tools, emotional support, and lobbying for better patient care and policy.

Resilience and the Human Spirit: The experiences of several individuals, including Avastin sufferers, provide witness to the human spirit's tenacity. We are motivated to tackle hardship with courage and optimism by the strength, hope, and tenacity exhibited by patients and their families. The knowledge gained from their experiences strengthens the conviction that a better future is achievable.

The Never-Ending Search for a Cure: Although we applaud the progress made in the treatment of cancer, finding a cure is still the top priority. Globally, scientists and activists are dedicated to discovering long-term treatments for cancer. This is an important objective that we are getting closer to as science and medicine advance.

The Message of Hope: We have a message of hope for the future of cancer treatment. The experiences and tales told in this book, such as the Avastin voyage, are only a small portion of a greater story of development, resiliency, and metamorphosis. The environment that we are seeing is dynamic and changing, giving cancer patients and their families unprecedented hope.

In summary, more individualized and potent treatments, more patient-centered care, and continuous progress toward a cure are all promising developments in the field of cancer treatment. The tenacious nature of cancer patients and the ceaseless endeavors of researchers and medical professionals serve as guiding lights that promise a bright future. We keep in mind that every step we take now is one closer to a better future for all cancer sufferers as we head into this new chapter.